Consultant Nursing
in
Mental Health

Consultant Nursing
in
Mental health

Edited by

Gary Wilshaw

Kingsham

First published in 2005
by Kingsham Press

Oldbury Complex
Marsh Lane
Easthampnett
Chichester, West Sussex
PO18 0JW
United Kingdom

www.kingshampress.com

© 2005, Gary Wilshaw

Typeset in AGaramond

Printed and bound by
RPM Print & Design
2–3 Spur Road
Chichester
W. Sussex

ISBN: 1-904235-38-7

British Library Cataloging in Publication Data
A catalogue record of this book is available from the British Library

Wilshaw, Gary

Contributors

Phil Barker PhD RN FRCN has been a psychiatric nurse and psychotherapist for almost 35 years. He was:

- Appointed as the UK's first Professor of Psychiatric Nursing Practice at the Medical School, *University of Newcastle* England (1993-2002)
- Elected a Fellow of the *Royal College of Nursing UK* in 1995
- Awarded the Red Gate Award for Distinguished Professors at the University of Tokyo in 2000
- Inducted as a Doctor of the University at *Oxford Brookes University*, England, in 2001.

He has published 16 books, 50 book chapters and over 150 academic and professional papers in international journals and has been Visiting Professor at several European and Australasian Universities. His two latest books – *A Textbook of Psychiatric and Mental Health Nursing* and *Breakthrough: Spirituality and Mental Health* (with Poppy Buchanan-Barker) was published in the summer of 2003.

Presently, he is Visiting Professor in Health Science at *Trinity College, Dublin.*

He is also a Director of *Slie Eile,* a therapeutic community for people with serious mental health problems in Cork, Ireland, and a Director of *Clan Unity*, the International Mental Health Recovery Consultancy based in Scotland, where he also offers a (free) private psychotherapy service.

Nick Bohannon RMN BA (Hons) MA is a senior lecturer in mental health nursing at the University of Central Lancashire where he has worked since 1999. Prior to that for three years he was contracted to the Ministry of Health in Kuwait as Senior Nurse Tutor with an internationally recruited management team. He has a background in multi-agency working and organisational development.

His current research activity is in the field of service user evaluations of mental health care, and service user involvement in the pre-registration education of professionals working in mental health services.

Adrian Childs – RMN RGN Dip.N (Lond) MSc is Deputy Chief Executive & Director of Nursing at the Newcastle, North Tyneside & Northumberland Mental Health NHS Trust.

He commenced his health service career as a support worker for older people with mental health problems in Dorset, and moved to Surrey to undertake both RMN and RGN training. Adrian's clinical experience is of working in acute and mental health settings and in general management across many areas of the country. He was the lead for the Northern & Yorkshire NHS Executive for the National Nursing Leadership Project and is Chair and lead for the National Mental Health Nursing Leadership Programme. He is currently a member of the national steering group for leadership in Dangerous and Severe Personality Disorders and a member of the Nursing Advisory and Development group for NIMH(E).

Sallie Cooper is a mother and grandmother. She has many years' experience of teaching music to children with special needs. She herself is an enthusiastic cellist.

In her spare time, she studies with the Open University, plays in two amateur orchestras, and is an active campaigner for human rights. She is also a keen photographer and enjoys reading twentieth century literature and poetry. She hopes one day to go back to teaching, this time training teachers with a pro-creativity and anti-labelling lobby!

When well enough, Sallie also works closely with her local Mental Health Trust in the provision and development of local services and is actively interested in national developments and issues in the field of Mental Health.

Mark Hardcastle RMN, BSc (Hons), Cert Ed (FE) ENB 650 & A48, is a Consultant Nurse in Acute Mental Health Care. He works for West Sussex Health and Social Care where he is the joint project local lead for the Sainsbury Centre for Mental Health Acute Solutions project, which aims to develop a new model of acute in-patient care. As a Modernisation Agency Associate he is enthusiastic in contributing to the recent debate about 'reshaping the role of the psychiatrist'.

His clinical expertise is based on 'giving a damn' about people, cognitive behaviour therapy and family work. Bad habits include Hull City, Morris dancing and Harvey's beer.

Steve Harrison RMN BSc (Hons) ENB 603,998 Dip CMH has been employed by Tees and North East Yorkshire Trust as a consultant nurse since September 2001. He works at the Newberry Centre for Young People with teenagers experiencing major mental health problems. His career started in 1979 as a nursing assistant in the local residential adolescent mental health unit. He qualified as a mental health nurse in 1983 and has subsequently pursued his interest in child and adolescent mental health.

Steve has undertaken a range of roles ranging from staff nurse to CPN, through to community team leader. Key achievements include contributing to the 1995 thematic review 'Together We Stand, developing community Child and Adolescent Mental Health services' in the South Tees area and, coordinating with his management colleagues, the relocation of CAMHS to the West Lane site in Middlesbrough where the new, purpose-built in-patient unit has been used as a model for service development for units in other areas. A graduate of

Teesside University, Steve is currently a part time lecturer on the Child and Adolescent Honours Degree pathway at the University of York.

Alongside his clinical commitments, current areas of development include the early intervention of psychosis team, the enhancement of outcome measures, and the development of the tier four clinical governance regional network. Steve also contributed to the Department of Health's National CAMHS Mapping Project.

Away from work, Steve supports and is supported by his wife and children, Middlesbrough Football Club and his co-contributors to Fly Me To The Moon, the local football club fanzine.

Nick Holdsworth BA, MA, RMN, is Consultant Nurse – Deliberate Self-harm at the Newcastle, North Tyneside & Northumberland Mental Health NHS Trust

He first worked in mental health care in the USA in the early 1980s and has been a mental health nurse in the North East of England for the past fifteen years. He has been Nurse Consultant in Deliberate Self-harm since April 2001. He has a record in research, development and associated publications and is an Honorary Senior Research Associate at the University of Northumbria, where he also teaches. He has led local policy developments in several areas associated with nursing research and practice development.

Mick Norman RMN, DipCPN, BA (Hons) undertook his RMN training at the Central Hospital, Warwick, from 1986 to 1989. After qualifying he moved to Oxford where from 1989 until 1998 he specialised in addictions work. During this time he worked on an in-patient detoxification unit with involvement in setting up a community-based low-threshold methadone project, as a Development Officer in addictions with Oxfordshire Probation Service, and for 6 years was a CPN in the Community Addictions Team. During this time he undertook the CPN Diploma on a secondment basis at Oxford Brookes University, with placements in Oxford's Elmore Community Support Team – a fore-runner of today's assertive outreach teams – and the Barnes Unit. In 1998 he was invited to work at the John Radcliffe Hospital, Oxford, in the Department of Psychological Medicine as a Clinical Nurse Specialist.

Mick moved to North Yorkshire in 1998 and for a year was a CPN in general adult psychiatry in the rural locality of Ryedale, followed by almost 2 years setting up and running an extension of the Scarborough based, Beacon award winning Mental Health Primary Care Team in the locality. Since 2002 he has been the Team Manager for the Ryedale CMHT and has collaborated with the editor on a number of mental health based projects as well as completing a BA (Hons) at York University.

In his spare time, he has for the past 2 years been attempting to complete the restoration of an 850cc Moto Guzzi motorcycle with distraction from a wife and 2-year-old son.

Tracy Packer has worked in the development of services for older people with a cognitive disability at North Bristol Trust since 1994. She has worked with older people who are acutely ill in hospital since 1990, when she qualified as a Registered General Nurse at University College Hospital, London. In April 2000, Tracy became one of the first Nurse Consultants in the country. This exciting opportunity has enabled her to continue her practice development work, with continued clinical experience in care settings that reflect the 'real world' of care.

Tracy is particularly interested in developing dementia care skills for individuals who work outside the mental health sector, but who still encounter people with dementia on a daily basis. Her clinical work presents her with a diverse range of needs and dilemmas, but she is particularly interested in the impact of the acute hospital environment upon the experience of care and future living choices.

In 1998, Tracy accompanied Professor Tom Kitwood to the USA to co-facilitate Dementia Care Mapping Courses, and is currently Licensed to train the Dementia Care Mapping Method at Basic and Advanced Level by Bradford Dementia Group in affiliation with Bradford University. More recently, Tracy was a guest of the Western Australian Alzheimer's Association, where she facilitated seminars for managers and staff of acute hospitals and care homes; as well as workshops for family carers and people with dementia. She has begun to publish her work widely and is the Consultant Care Practice Editor for the Journal of Dementia Care. Tracy is a Visiting Research Fellow at the University of the West of England, and in March 2001, was appointed onto the Department of Health Standing Nursing & Midwifery Advisory Committee.

Geoff Speight, MA, RMN, RGN, DPSN, CPN.Cert, FETC, currently works as Senior lecturer in the Department of Nursing at the University of Central Lancashire. His main teaching responsibilities are on both Pre and post registration courses. Community mental health nursing along with Mental Health Law, Policy and Ethics are his main areas of teaching. Prior to this he worked for more years than he cares to recall as a community mental health nurse and CMHT co-ordinator in the Blackpool area.

He has an abiding interest in the history of mental health care and believes that mental nurses could do worse than revisit the work of the moral treatment pioneers. He also feels that the original concept of the provision of 'asylum' is one that mental health services should embrace, alongside complementary efforts to support recovery.

A long time cyclist and tandemist he has recently taken up the motorised version.

Ian Trodden RMN BA (Hons) BSc (ENB 650) qualified as a mental health nurse in 1987. Following this he has worked in a variety of mental health settings including acute in-patient, sub-acute and community services.

In 1990, Ian left nursing to embark full time on a BA (Hons) in social sciences at Nottingham University, graduating in 1993. He then returned to nursing where once again he worked mainly in the acute in-patient environment, and later with a community team. He has a BSc (Hons/first class) in Cognitive Behavioural Psychotherapy.

Ian later worked within a psychology service as a Cognitive Behavioural Therapist, and continued – within this role- to work closely within the acute in-patient and community services. He secured his first post as a Consultant Nurse within the acute in-patient setting (north locality) at Tees and North East Yorkshire Trust.

In the two years in this capacity, Ian has established the Trust wide acute care forum, initiated an enhanced skills training course for all staff working within the acute in patient setting. Along with a colleague, he was commissioned to introduce Psycho-social interventions for the Western Health Board in Ireland.

Ian has presented at both national and local conferences, and organised conferences including one addressing nursing leadership that attracted renowned speakers in this field. Other interests include user, carer and advocacy leadership training, which has led to the development of a programme attracting interest across the UK.

He enjoys watching rugby (he used to play but is now to old!), football (Liverpool FC) reading and socialising with family and friends.

Lyn Williams RMN; Dip. H.E; HNC Public Admin; is Consultant Nurse, Liaison Psychiatry with Tees & North East Yorkshire NHS Trust.

Lyn qualified as an RMN 1992, and then worked within acute inpatient admission areas for elderly mentally ill and acute general psychiatry. She began working in Liaison Psychiatry in 1996 when this function was first established in Middlesbrough.

As part of her M.Sc. Health Science dissertation, she is currently undertaking research looking at patients admitted to hospital with non-specific chest pain. Here, she is looking at 'costs' involved and the potential benefits of joint physical and mental health assessment on admission for this patient group.

Within her Consultant Nurse role, she has developed partnership working within Cancer Care at the local Acute Trust. She has initiated a nurse to nurse fast-track referral route for mental health assessment for patients diagnosed with breast cancer and presenting mental health problems. Her other current key areas of interest are integrated care pathway development for those people presenting with deliberate self-harm, suicide prevention, and competency development for staff in Liaison psychiatry work.

Gary Wilshaw PhD, MA, BSc(Hons), RMN, RGN, DipN (Lond), DipCPN, CertEd. is Consultant Nurse, Primary & Community Nursing for the Tees & North East Yorkshire NHS Trust, based in Scarborough. He is also the Head of

Nursing for the North-East Yorkshire Locality of the Trust, and visiting Senior Lecturer at the University of York, and a freelance psychotherapist.

His key interests and publications include primary mental health care, the integration of psycho-therapeutic approaches, access to psychological therapies, qualitative research in healthcare, suicide prevention and creative therapies. He has a special interest in Cognitive Analytic Therapy (CAT). His PhD research mapped the development of effective therapeutic relationships between nurses and their patients. He is a reviewer for the Journal of Advanced Nursing and external examiner for two British University Departments of Nursing.

Over his 30 year working life, Gary has held senior practice, educational and managerial posts in 'general' and mental health nursing – in addition to working also in the private sector. He was Head of Division of Mental Health at the University of Central Lancashire until taking up his Consultant Nurse post in 2001.

Adam Wilshaw BA (Hons) PGCE read English and American Literature at the University of Manchester. He is now pursuing a career in journalism.

Acknowledgements

I am greatly indebted to all contributors for their creativity, work, ideas, willingness and enthusiasm. In addition, the support of Tees & NE Yorkshire NHS Trust has proved tireless and an example of the constructive and encouraging style of this organisation.

I am also grateful to the publishers for their encouragement, and to Anand Kumar in particular, for supporting the original idea and making a challenging process much easier than it might have been.

Finally, my thanks go to Elaine for her continued patience, encouragement, love and support.

Contents

Preface

The NHS is changing rapidly. We now have the most comprehensive policy framework in the history of the NHS including the National Service Framework for mental health. The resources being made available are at a higher level than ever before – double the rate of growth previously experienced. The long-term relative decline of the NHS has been halted and it is becoming possible to improve and extend services.

However it will not be possible to meet the needs and demands of the people we serve if we go on working in traditional ways. More resources and a national policy framework are not enough. It is essential that we do things differently based on two fundamental principles – the needs of patients, clients and carers *and* the skills knowledge and experience of the people – the staff – of the NHS.

Traditional methods of service delivery have sought to confine NHS staff to roles dictated by tradition and professional boundaries. Unless tradition is challenged we will not liberate the enormous potential of the people in the NHS and we will not meet the needs of the people we serve.

Consultant Nurses are at the forefront of the changes that need to be made. At last it is possible for nurses to enhance and apply their skills, knowledge and experience in the development of new services, roles and relationships.

Nurses have always been the foundation and cornerstone of the NHS. Now Consultant Nurses are building on those foundations to demonstrate what nurses can do, given the opportunity and freedom from the constraints of tradition and demarcation.

Leadership is about showing the way by 'going first'. Consultant Nurses are demonstrating leadership in action and making it more likely that the new NHS will respond to the needs and demands of patients, clients and carers.

Ken Jarrold CBE
Chief Executive
County Durham and Tees Valley Strategic Health Authority

Introduction

Gary Wilshaw

This book is the product of a collaboration that began in December 2001, shortly after I took up my first Consultant Nurse post. I was lucky to become part of an NHS Trust that had identified the potential of the nascent role and had invested in the creation of five posts (now seven) in the sub-specialities of primary care, liaison, forensic, acute and child & adolescent mental health. My colleagues and I have spent two years developing the roles in ways that reflect local needs and priorities, national guidelines, national thinking and international opinion. These two years, which have been profoundly rewarding in a number of ways, have thrown up enormous challenges. In one way this book is an attempt to get to grips with some of them.

The specification offered in Making a Difference: Strengthening the Nursing, Midwifery and Health Visiting contribution to Health and Healthcare (DoH, 1999) sets out the core ambitions for this new role. However these guidelines must not stand in isolation. While serving an absolutely necessary function, we should not let guidelines impose limitations on our exploration of this new territory. Just as an explorer in uncharted lands must look beyond a given indistinct and untested route and pencil in their own additions to an elementary map, so too the incumbent Consultant Nurse is required to be bold and brave if they wish to look upon new horizons. This exploration has led to a period of significant creative development, with different and at times competing ideas and dynamics informing the shaping of the contours of this work. National networks of Consultant Nurses have emerged and meet regularly to share ideas and to develop a vision of the future where Consultant Nurses play a key role in developing services fit for the twenty-first century.

This book is a reflection of these times and dynamics. It is born of optimism, excitement and a great challenge. At best, the role would appear to satisfy the long-awaited need for a model of clinically oriented leadership posts. This is quite distinct from the essential elements of the general management model, which by definition makes no claims to clinical wisdom and yet has directed much clinical activity since the mid nineteen-eighties. The 'general' in general management, whilst being its strength in terms of managerial accountability for whole services, is also its weakness when it comes to the setting of clinical direction based on clinical *intelligence*. Alongside medical, and other Consultant colleagues, the Consultant Nurse role can provide insight to services and thus promote a form of planning and action that is more attuned to patient and practitioner alike.

This Consultant role is also, by definition, able to bring a unique *nursing* perspective, by reminding healthcare systems that it is the *patients' experience* of their distress that is the proper focus for attention. The Consultant Nurse has perhaps a unique position of authority from which to support nurses in doing what they do best – to provide a sense of fellowship with the patient and a relationship within which human suffering can be acknowledged, shared and contained. It is only from this position that truly helpful and collaborative work with the patient can emerge. It is intended that the contents of this book will support a discussion of these ideas, and the ways in which the role of Consultant Nurse can help services maintain and enhance the degree to which they focus on patient experience (as opposed to the 'measures', judgements, or opinions of others).

For these seeds of hopes to come to fruition however, employers must address not just the *recruitment* of suitable people, but also the infrastructure to exploit the role and the personal talents of incumbents to the maximum once they *are* secured. Post holders need support, access to continued development and most of all – a 'public' recognition and sanctioning of authority and agency within the organisation. It is not enough to expect that post-holders will 'win' the respect that authority is built upon. Winning the respect of colleagues in this way is fine in terms of the development of one's transformational leadership function. However, employers also need to give sufficient thought to how the post integrates with existing chains of communication and authority, and they should be willing to *change* existing systems if needed.

The majority of this book is – very deliberately – written by Consultant Nurses. It is also supported by chapters from others who have a specific perspective on the role and its potential. The latter group includes a highly respected health care leader and Chief Executive of a Strategic Health Authority (Ken Jarold); an inspirational and influential scholar, author, practitioner and teacher in mental health nursing (Phil Barker); a service user with a great deal of wisdom to share about her experiences of mental health care (Sallie Cooper); a highly respected and grounded Community Mental Health Team leader (Mick Norman); two practice-rooted academics with special interests in mental healthcare organisational development (Geoff Speight and Nick Bohannon); and finally a senior manager and mental health leading-light, whose foresight and energy has been instrumental in the creation of a significant critical mass of Consultant Nurse posts in the North of England (Adrian Childs).

I have briefly explored the purpose of this book with reference to the broad issues that have driven the thinking behind the enterprise as a whole. I would like now to examine how, more specifically, the chapters address one or more of the so called 'key functions' of the Consultant Nurse role as spelled out by the Department of Health in 1999. These are a clinical expertise function; leadership; practice development and education/research.

Adrian Childs maps the policy developments and initiatives that have led to the creation of the Consultant Nurse role. In addition, he clearly sets out the expectations of the post holders and clarifies some of the key political dynamics and power bases shaping mental health care both in an historical and a contemporary sense. Adrian's analysis of the importance of nursing leadership, at this time of revolution in health-care, is timely. His reference to the concept of *servant leadership* (Giampetro, Meyer *et al.*, 1998) complements **Mick Norman**'s idea that the Consultant Nurse in mental health may have a critical function to play in *enabling* the work of other mental health nurses. His assertion is that there is a helpful parallel between the way the mental health nurse engages (or fails to engage) with the patient, and the way the Consultant engages (or fails to engage) with other professionals and services as a whole. The support and the *challenge* offered to nursing to maintain and enhance its standards is the focus of a chapter by **Steve Harrison**. Steve makes the case for a redressing of the balance between the challenges and support offered to nurses, and he examines the part the Consultant Nurse can play in this process.

The theme of leadership is further developed by **Lyn Williams** and **Nick Bohannon** who investigate the possibilities of 'clinically intelligent leadership' as modelled by Consultant Nursing at its best. Lyn and Nick offer a useful perspective on the dynamics of the power and control of healthcare, and their chapter also exists as an interesting companion to **Mark Hardcastle**'s chapter. Mark provides vital advice for Consultant Nurses considering entering the waters/politics of healthcare.

Adam Wilshaw's interview with **Tracy Packer** offers more than just insight into a typical working week. What this chapter illustrates is the enormous scope and demand of the busy schedule and the broad, systemic relevance of the Consultant role (as reflected in **Gary Wilshaw**'s thoughts on 'abstraction and impact'). Tracy gives a practical illustration of the service development, leadership and educational functions in the broadest sense. In a more particular way, **Ian Trodden** provides a practical illustration of the use of a specific therapeutic model (Cognitive Behavioural Therapy) as the basis for practice development initiatives in an acute in-patient setting. His work reminds us of the role of outcome orientation that many will value as a feature of constructive and goal oriented professional helping.

A key theme that is illustrated in the contributions by **Phil Barker**, **Sallie Cooper**, **Gary Wilshaw** and **Geoff Speight** can be summarised as an analysis of caring and the relevance of this deceptively simple term to the emerging Consultant Nurse mindset. This theme is central to the book as a whole, taking on as it does the assertion that the role has 'expert practice' at its core, and then asking (a) what does 'expert practice' mean? (b) are there any conflicts in the quest to be 'experts', and yet *remain* nurses? (c) is it possible to re-define *expertise* from a uniquely *nursing* perspective? and (d) is it possible to avoid the pitfalls of seduction by the psycho-technologies, and the risks of increased distance from the essential humanity and *ordinariness* of many of the most helpful interactions that seem to make human suffering more tolerable?

The final theme found in the chapters of this book is most clearly focused in the contributions of **Nick Holdsworth** and **Gary Wilshaw** who explore some of the considerations facing the Consultant Nurse during the fulfilment of their research role requirements and ambitions. In addition to some considerations of the choices in methodology, attention is drawn to the sometimes ignored rigour with which *qualitative* methods can be applied. It is suggested here that such methods can offer a valuable and practical approach to learning about working with *people*.

Consultant Nurse or Nurse Consultant?

Throughout this book, the term Consultant Nurse is preferred to that of Nurse Consultant. This choice is a reflection of decisions made by post-holders across the country to opt for this title as a better reflection of the ambitions of the role. The Consultant Nurse title is more equitable with Consultant grades of other professions (one rarely hears of a Psychiatrist Consultant) and places appropriate emphasis on the *Consultation* function available to *all* in the healthcare economy.

Patients, clients, service users, customers or ... people?

As Phil barker points out in his chapter, it is easy to be distracted by a debate about the most appropriate way to refer to those whom we set out to help. In this book I have chosen to use the term 'patient' more or less throughout, for reasons that I shall continue to reflect on long after this book is published. It may be that I am just truly bored with the political correctness that has dogged this debate for decades. I feel I must acknowledge the evidence of my experience and accept that most people I have attempted to work with or help in my professional capacity have either wished, expected or preferred to be thought of as 'patient'. Or it may be that I find, as I grow older, that I am increasingly comfortable with the idea of 'patiency'. The term conjures up a powerful and potentially positive element of the (often rightly) much-criticised 'medical model': that it can be enormously reassuring to be cared for by someone whom one can trust because of their professionalism. The term also perhaps signals a dynamic that *allows* for a temporary relinquishing of autonomy by the individual in care that may be *needed, wished for* and at times entirely appropriate. I believe that to allow for such a temporary relinquishment of autonomy is congruent with the best ambitions of nursing and that it may be even be the ultimate act of compassion.

CHAPTER ONE

The making of the Consultant Nurse

Adrian Childs

Introduction

The development of nursing is seen as an integral part of modernising the National Health Service (NHS). Indeed the Consultant Nurse has been heralded outside the nursing profession as a new clinical leader able to play a significant part in delivering the Government's radical change programme for the NHS. The ten-year strategic plan for the NHS, *The NHS Plan – A Plan for Investment, a Plan for Reform* (DoH 2000), clearly articulates a role for Consultant Nurses in developing clinical and referral protocols. This chapter will endeavour to explore some of the roots of the Consultant Nurse role and identify a number of the influencing factors that have led to the development of such a key post.

The Consultant Nurse role

The role of the Consultant Nurse was first described in the national nursing strategy, *Making a Difference – Strengthening the Nursing, Midwifery and Health Visiting Contribution to Health and Healthcare* (DoH 1999). The post was described as being part of a new career structure for nursing, part of a career trajectory from Health Care Assistant to Consultant Practitioner. It was anticipated that these new roles would provide opportunities for experienced and expert nurses to work at a senior level within the health service and enable them to remain in clinical practice.

In the autumn of 1999 the Department of Health produced detailed guidance which identified how these new posts were to be established, the aim of which was to ensure consistency across the country (NHS Executive 1999). It is suggested within this guidance that the role of the

Consultant Nurse was created by the Government in order to address several concerns that had been articulated by the nursing profession. Among these concerns were the limitations of the nursing career structure – the most experienced and expert nurses leaving practice-based posts to advance their careers and improve their earnings and the need to strengthen professional leadership. These new posts, it was reported (NHS Executive 1999), would help to provide better outcomes for patients by improving services and quality, would strengthen leadership and provide a new career opportunity and help retain experienced and expert nurses in clinical practice.

In order to achieve these outcomes the guidance separated the role into four primary functions:

1. Expert practice
2. Professional leadership and consultancy
3. Education, training and development
4. Practice and service development, research and evaluation.

It was anticipated that the posts could be established in all areas of health care delivery. The weight attributable to each of the four primary functions, and the time spent in undertaking them, was to be determined by the creators of the posts. However the guidance is very clear that at least 50% of the Consultant Nurse's time must be spent working in clinical practice with patients, clients or communities. This, the guidance suggests, ensures practitioners are able to maintain professional competence and professional expertise.

An historical perspective

It is perhaps simplistic to accept that the Consultant Nurse role was developed purely to meet the demands of the healthcare agenda of the 21st century. One only has to look back at nursing history to realise that Florence Nightingale was delivering nursing care, in what she described as organised concepts with a social relevance distinct from medicine. She was attempting to significantly influence healthcare delivery through leadership. Moreover, she insisted that effective nurses possessed skills, character and discipline (Nightingale 1969) all of which can be seen in the prescribed role of the Consultant Nurse – skills to deliver the required clinical care, character to act as a leader of nurses and nursing practice and discipline to deliver the current healthcare agenda.

Nightingale is not the only proponent of a stronger nursing voice. Attempts have been made in recent years to create a more influential profession. Shaw (1993) suggests that one of the strengths of the nursing profession has been its consistency in identifying its boundaries and domain. Salmon (1966) endeavoured to provide a nursing career structure that enabled nurses to move from a bedside, clinical role to a management role through a progressive hierarchy, thus extending the boundaries of the previous nursing remit. What this hierarchy achieved was exactly the *opposite* of what is required of the Consultant Nurse – it removed nurses from a clinical into a managerial role and, because they were not all adequately prepared for this new role, the structure became increasingly more unstable (Welford 2002).

Griffiths (1983) developed what was believed to be an antidote to this instability in the general management structure. His model devolved responsibility and brought with it corporate decision-making. Doctors, who up until this time, had made decisions based on clinical judgements alone now had to account to general managers and were therefore only one part of the decision-making process. However, little account was taken of the nursing profession within this structure, and nurses were forced to make stark choices. Many left nursing and entered a career in general management. Although this may have been recognised in the production of *A Strategy For Nursing* (DoH 1989), which identified a clear need for leadership within nursing, there was little demonstrable evidence in the clinical environment.

What becomes evident from considering the past is that nurses and nursing have not been able to secure the career structure or recognition of the contribution they make to healthcare that they clearly deserve. To achieve such goals requires a fundamental examination of the factors that will enable nursing to play a central role in health care delivery.

The power to succeed

Aziz (2000) suggests that nursing has compared itself to the medical profession for some time, and although nursing practice has developed significantly, nurses have continued to emulate doctors. This is perhaps due to the fact that doctors are perceived to have more influence over patient care and the way in which health care is delivered (Aziz, 2000). The development of the Consultant Nurse roles can then be considered as one way to empower the nursing profession and enable it to be seen as central to the health care agenda.

Power and empowerment are intrinsically linked. However, they are frequently seen as being at opposite ends of a continuum, thus presenting an apparent dichotomy. Empowerment is seen as an abstract concept that has positive connotations: it is a dynamic and sharing process in which power can be given away and taken over, but is also seen as something that can benefit organisations, individuals and communities (Kuokkanen & Leino-Kilpi 2000). Power itself is generally perceived as being negative and is associated with hierarchical structures, with one person being able to limit or restrict the actions of another. Kuokkanen & Leino-Kilpi (2000) suggest that power is extrapersonal in that it is not purely something that comes from within the individual. An increase in power for one person has to be compensated for by a decrease in the power of another.

A more positive view of power is that described by Kanter (1979) who suggests that power could be seen as providing efficacy and goal orientation. Kanter (1979) asserts that organisations in themselves do not exert power, it is generated by individuals within the organisation and does not necessarily relate to the hierarchical structure. The building blocks upon which power is generated are the creation of opportunities, effective information and support.

A more complex view of power is provided by Foucault (1991), who believes that power and knowledge are inextricably linked. Therefore, where there is knowledge there is also power. He believes that we are able to increase the amount of power we possess by increasing our knowledge. This suggests that power is not necessarily bestowed upon individuals, or groups, but can be earned and can also be exercised to a greater or lesser extent in differing situations. Turner (1987) supports this view and believes that absolute power does not exist. Power may be in existence in particular circumstances but may be very limited in others and he suggests that this will depend upon the roles that are assumed and the ability, character and status of the individual or group.

When considering these views power should not be seen purely as an action or the ability to control or dominate a situation or an argument. The exercising of power requires subtle skills including the ability to manipulate thoughts, to persuade and to influence attitudes and social relationships. It is therefore essential that those who assume power must accept the responsibilities that go with it in order for it to be a beneficial and positive tool for the development of nursing.

Power and empowerment are closely linked. However, to assume that delegating power empowers individuals and groups is perhaps an under-estimation. Rappaport (1984) suggests that empowerment should be seen as a mechanism, a process by which individuals, organisations and communities are able to gain a sense of mastery over their own lives. This suggests that empowerment is a developmental process, something that cannot be given but needs to evolve. Empowerment can be seen as a useful umbrella concept that can be used to describe professional development within the nursing profession. Empowerment is then a process of influence and power sharing. Empowerment focuses on motivation and commitment to drive forward.

Du Plat-Jones (1999) believes that not only is there a strong linkage between power and empowerment but that poor representation is also linked to a lack of power. In terms of representation she suggests that social judgement is among the methods that can be used to enhance power. Nursing has, in the past, relied on a public image that is stereotypical, that of 'nursing angels', that does not accurately reflect the developments and expertise of the modern day profession. In accepting this social judgement nursing has allowed the skills and expertise of the profession to become devalued, especially when considered against the other healthcare professions. Du Plat-Jones (1999) insists, therefore, that nursing must raise its profile and society's opinion in order to gain power, and empower the profession.

Influence through politics

To date much of the focus for empowering the nursing profession has been on developing nursing practice. Although this has improved the quality of patient care, it has done little to enable the profession to influence the development of health policy. The result of this has been a poor relationship between nursing and health policy. Indeed Robinson (1991) suggested that the nursing profession operated in a political vacuum, with health policy being developed with minimal input from nurses, except when it came to implementation.

In a study by Antrobus and Kitson (1999) nursing leaders were considered in terms of four areas: the development of clinical nursing, executive roles, academic roles and politics. They argued that in order to make a significant contribution to the development of health care policy, nursing must begin to function within a political environment. The study also suggests that many nursing leaders perform a translation and interpretation role in order to bridge the gap between policy and nursing practice. They found it necessary to use alternative language in nursing in order for nurses to understand what was required of them. The nursing profession exacerbates the gap between policy and practice by employing ideologies and using language that is different policy speak, which leaves them powerless within the political arena. This results in nursing not being clearly understood and therefore not considered to be a priority in developing healthcare policy. In order to rectify this position, nursing must move away from an introspective professional stance and begin to function within the wider political processes.

In the past many nurses have not considered politics to be their concern. However, it is difficult to see how they are able to distance themselves when they are required to deliver care and treatment according to policies developed through central government. Northway (1996) believes that nurses must become more politically aware and challenge existing power structures if they are to really influence healthcare.

Traditionally nursing has been considered to be a form of service work and therefore was not seen as a political force. This view has been reinforced by the large number of females employed within the profession (Northway 1996). Robinson (1991) believes this strongly to be the case but suggests that other barriers within the profession also reduce its political force. Throughout nursing history, divisions within the profession have existed. Vertical divisions have been highlighted between nurses in clinical practice and nurses who hold management positions, but in more recent times divisions have developed horizontally, across the profession between specialisms. These divisions have proved difficult to manage and, rather than coming together and recognising the diversity within the profession, nursing has remained divided and been unable to successfully capitalise on the common interests and concerns that could generate the move towards political participation.

Northway (1996) also suggests that traditional views and definitions present barriers to political participation. The public perception of nurses as 'nursing angels' (Du Plat-Jones 1999) can be seen as a form of control over the profession, in that society has given it a status and therefore determined how much power and privilege it is able to exercise. In accepting these societal definitions and values, nursing has also accepted that it has a place within society from where it is unable to move, thus limiting its political influence. In order to gain a more influential role within healthcare, nursing must reflect on the public's perceptions and redefine its current role.

Expert practice

For nursing to play a greater role in health care, it must develop a more political approach. Mullally (2001) believes that this is not merely about increasing professional power. Politics in nursing is about influence and exercising that influence to shape and develop healthcare policy and practice at both a local and national level. It is important to note that no single profession is able to do this alone and therefore an inclusive approach needs to be maintained. Nursing needs to create relationships with other health care professions and work in partnership, recognising that a collaborative approach will enable the exercising of influence.

A critical aspect of influence is credibility, and Mullally (2001) suggests that this is based on knowledge and expertise, much of which is grounded in the nurse's ability to deliver expert nursing practice. Expert nursing practice has also been described as 'advanced nursing practice' and Pearson & Peels (2002) suggest it has always existed in nursing, and has increasingly developed since nurses began to undertake medical tasks during the 1990s. The core elements of advanced nursing practice sit comfortably with the role of the Consultant Nurse in that they include: clinical activity, research, teaching, consultancy and leadership.

Hamric and Spross (1989) consider advanced nursing practice and describe primary criteria and competencies. Advanced nurse practitioners should be educated at masters level or above with a specific area of practice that enables them to demonstrate expert clinical practice. They should be professionally accredited in their specialist area and their practice skills should not only be concerned with patients but also the wider sphere of families, carers and the community. However, with such a broad scope of inclusion, it is easy to recognise why nursing has had such difficulties in agreeing upon what advanced nursing practice is and how it can be recognised.

There is also confusion between specialist nursing practice and advanced nursing practice both within and outside of the profession. Hamric and Spross (1989) believe that specialist nurses, employing specialist nursing practice, work at a post registration level in a defined specialist area. However, Davies and Hughes (2002), while suggesting that there is a difference between the two levels of practice, state that advance nursing practice is used to describe the functioning of the Clinical Nurse Specialist's role. Davies and Hughes (2002) argue that the difference between specialist and advanced nursing practice results from the variation in the individual's knowledge and skills level and is based on experience and educational preparation.

One of the ways the nursing profession has attempted to distinguish between these two levels of practice is to create roles that reflect different functions, for instance Clinical Nurse Specialist, Nurse Practitioner (Davies and Hughes 2002). However, Davies and Hughes (2002) warn that there is potential to create divisiveness within the profession by doing so. An added complication has been that the profession has introduced these roles across the country without congruency, resulting in a plethora of titles and roles that do not reflect any marked difference between specialist and advanced nursing practice.

Perhaps a more productive view of advanced nursing practice is to consider the main characteristics of it and how it is delivered, thus suggesting that it is the role that is different rather than the practice itself. Patterson and Haddard (1992) clearly articulate this in that they consider advanced nursing practice to be characterised by risk taking, vision, flexibility, the ability to articulate clearly, inquisitiveness and leading. Combining these characteristics with the competencies of: clinical expertise, critical thinking and analysis, clinical judgement, decision making, leadership and management communication, problem solving, collaboration and education and research (Davies and Hughes 2002) firmly places advanced nursing practice in a role. It is clinical expertise combined with these high level attributes that differentiates specialist nursing practice and advanced nursing practice.

The critical issues around advanced nursing practice are therefore how it can be clearly defined, how it is regulated and how it can be recognised not only by the nursing profession but also the wider health care community. The overriding goal is to develop nursing practice, and the profession, to meet the changing needs of society. In implementing advanced nursing practice Carroll (2002) warns against creating elitism within the profession and that the skills and qualities of advanced nurse practitioners should be determined nationally. The guidance produced to implement the role of the Consultant Nurse (NHS Executive 1999) aims to ensure there is national congruency and clearly describes the skills and qualities required for such a post. The guidance also infers that this is a new role in nursing and perhaps therefore needs to be somewhat elitist in order to compete with the current dominant professions of the NHS.

The need for effective leadership

The congruency required across the country cannot be achieved without developing a culture within the profession where there is a consistent philosophy and shared professional values. The development of this culture within the profession needs to be effectively communicated and supported and can only be achieved with effective leadership. McMillan and Conway (2002) suggest that nursing leaders are those individuals who cause us to rethink the concepts we have of what it means to be a nurse, to manage, educate and research and to consider how we enact our nursing roles. Leadership in nursing is about directing change. Indeed, Mullally (2001) suggests that in order to deliver the health care agenda, nursing requires transformation and that this can only be achieved with effective leadership. We must develop nurses who are able to motivate, challenge processes, inspire others and be prepared to take calculated risks.

Leadership is frequently confused with managing and in the past it has been associated with titles and status. However, there is a growing movement that considers leadership to be more about a set of behaviours that aim towards the achievement of specific ends, rather than stating how to attain those specific goals. Within nursing there is a moral dimension to leadership, in that the ends we pursue and the means by which they are achieved must be congruent with the ethics, morals and values of the profession (Mullally 2001).

Giampetro Meyer and others (1998) identify a number of leadership models including transformational, transactional and servant leadership. Transformational leadership concerns itself with those who are able to inspire others by articulating a clear vision and promoting change. Transactional leaders tend to consider leadership as an exchange process: in that if you give you will receive something in return. Servant leadership is perhaps a more complex concept in that the priorities of the servant leader are the complex needs of their employees. Servant leaders have a genuine concern for others. They too strive for continuous development and improvement through collaboration and coaching, they inspire and influence but are also consistent in their approach. It is through this type of leadership model that complex matrix organisations are developed, where leaders are influential beyond their immediate surroundings.

Antrobus and Kitson (1999) suggest that nursing leaders, regardless of level, combine their sphere of influence with clinical practice in that the knowledge they have from clinical practice is instrumental to their thinking as nursing leaders. They also believe that as the majority of nurses work within a traditional direct care-giving environment the populist view is that nurses are concerned with operational issues and not those of strategic or policy development. It is therefore essential that nursing strives to develop roles and mechanisms that enable individuals to work within both the domains of clinical practice and policy development.

Conclusion

The NHS Plan (DoH 2000) sets out the agenda for the reform of the NHS and nursing features as integral part of the Government's plan to modernise healthcare delivery. Throughout history the nursing profession has attempted to develop and maintain a dynamic purpose. Florence Nightingale (1969) believed that nursing had to progress; and that not to do so was to go backwards. Much has been achieved in developing clinical practice. However, the impact of nursing on a broader front has been less successful.

The Consultant Nurse role has been developed to assist in delivering the Government's agenda. Furthermore, it is a vehicle to enable the nursing profession to influence the way in which healthcare policy is developed and implemented. The fundamental components of the role are an accumulation of those aspects of nursing that the profession has struggled in pulling together. Authors have suggested that the profession does not look to our medical colleagues in developing these roles (Welford 2000; Castledine 1999) however doctors have been extremely successful in influencing healthcare decisions though a combination of their power and clinical expertise. It is perhaps shortsighted not to at least consider what elements have enabled them to be so powerful and learn from them.

In order to influence the development and implementation of healthcare policy, nursing needs to be involved in the political arena. As a profession nursing is somewhat politically naïve; nursing needs to understand its own historical and political context. The Consultant Nurse role has the opportunity to achieve this by working at a senior level and becoming involved in the political processes of everyday healthcare delivery.

A significant part of the Consultant Nurse's role is in clinical practice. It is clear that these nurses are expected to be expert practitioners. However, the debate within the profession continues about what advanced nursing practice, and therefore expert practice, is and how it is demonstrated. It is perhaps more important to consider how this advanced nursing practice is delivered: the expert practitioner is embodied within a role rather than defined through the particular clinical tasks it performs. The Consultant Nurse is a role that combines a number of skills including risk taking, influencing, clinical judgement and decision-making in order to provide the expert practitioner.

Finally, the nursing profession has long talked about the need for sound leadership. Leadership has been seen as something that is attached to a post of seniority and was seldom considered a requirement of clinical nurses. Leaders need to be able to challenge the status quo and seek better ways of doing things and they are required at all levels of the profession. However, those in senior leadership positions have a responsibility to set the tone and culture of organisations. These new Consultant Nurse roles have the opportunity to set that tone and culture not only for individual organisations but also for the profession itself.

References

Antrobus, S. and Kitson, A. (1999) Nursing Leadership: influencing and shaping health policy and nursing practice. *Journal of Advanced Nursing*, 29(3), pp. 746–757.

Aziz, B. (2000) Educating the doctors. *Nursing Management*, 7(2), pp. 30–31.

Carroll, M. (2002) Advanced nursing practice. *Nursing Standard*, 16(29), pp. 33–35.

Castledine, G. (1999) Nursing must be at the core of Consultant Nurses' work. *British Journal of Nursing*, 8(14), p. 966.

Davies, B. and Hughes, A.M. (2002) Clarification of advanced nursing practice: characteristics and competencies. *Clinical Nurse Specialist*, 16(3), pp. 147–152.

Department of Health (1989) *A Strategy for Nursing*. London: HMSO.

Department of Health (1999) *Making a Difference- Strengthening the Nursing, Midwifery and Health Visiting Contribution to Health and Healthcare*. London: Department of Health.

Department of Health (2000) *The NHS Plan: A Plan for Investment, a Plan for Reform*. Norwich: The Stationery Office.

Du Plat-Jones, J. (1999) Power and representation in nursing: a literature review. *Nursing Standard*, 13(49), pp. 39–42.

Foucault, M. (1991) *Discipline and Punish*. Penguin, Harmondsworth.

Giampetro Meyer, A., Brown, T., Browne, M.N., Kubaseck, N. (1998) Do we really need more leaders in business? *Journal of Business Ethics*, 17(15), pp. 1727–1736.

Griffiths, R. (1983) *NHS Management Enquiry*. London: DHSS.

Hamric, A. and Spross, J. (eds) (1989) *The Clinical Nurse Specialist in Theory and Practice*, 2nd edn. W.B. Saunders: Toronto.

Kanter, R. (1979) Power failure in management circuits. *Harvard Business Review*, 4, pp. 65–75.

Kuouuanen, L. and Leino-Kilpi, H. (2000) Power and empowerment in nursing: three theoretical approaches. *Journal of Advanced Nursing*, 31(1), pp. 235–241.

McMillan, M. and Conway, J. (2002) Exploring nursing leadership. *Australian Journal of Advanced Nursing*, 19(4), pp. 5–6.

Mullally, S. (2001) Leadership and politics. *Nursing Management*, 8(4), pp. 21–27.

NHS Executive (1999) Nurse, midwife and health visitor consultants. Establishing posts and making appointments. HSC 1999/217.

Nightingale, F. (1969) *Notes on Nursing: What It Is and What It Is Not*. Dover: New York.

Northway, R. (1996) Proceed with political care. *Nursing Management*, 3(3), pp. 14–15.

Patterson, C. and Haddad, B. (1992) The advanced nurse practitioner: common attributes. *Canadian Journal of Nursing Administration*, 5(3), pp. 18–22.

Pearson, A. and Peels, S. (2002) Advanced practice in nursing: international perspective. *International Journal of Nursing Practice*, 8(2), pp. S1–S4.

Rappaport, J. (1984) Studies in empowerment: introduction to the issue. *Prevention in Human Services*, 3, pp. 1–7.

Robinson, J. (1991) Power, politics and policy analysis in nursing. In Perry, A., Jolley, M. (eds) *Nursing, A Knowledge Base for Practice*. London: Edward Arnold.

Salmon, B. (1966) *Report of the Committee on Senior Nursing Staff Structure*. London: HMSO.

Shaw, M. (1993) The discipline of nursing: historical roots, current perspectives, future directions. *Journal of Advanced Nursing*, 18, pp. 1651–1656.

Turner, B. (1987) *Medical Power and Social Knowledge*. Sage: London.

Welford, C. (2002) Matching theory to practice. *Nursing Management*, 9(4), pp. 7–11.

CHAPTER TWO

On the ward and around the world:
A week in the life of Tracy Packer, Consultant Nurse

Adam Wilshaw

'If I wasn't being challenging I would wonder if I was doing my job properly'

Tracy Packer, Consultant Nurse in Dementia Care

A large case-load

With more generosity than is usual – ten days notice rather than, say, two – the Department of Health announce they are to pay a visit. Figures and statistics will need to be collated and analysed in time for their arrival. Tracy Packer, Consultant Nurse in Dementia Care, will spend Monday morning working with her secretary in order to compile admission and discharge rates, the average age of patients, where patients come from, and where they go when they leave. The DoH will want to see a detailed profile of the current service-user group, and will be particularly interested in how this has changed (or not) since their last visit. Although Tracy Packer has invited this particular visit, the Trust has a 'no-star' rating and is under immense pressure. Questions must be anticipated. Why *should* older people with dementia have a service in the acute trust rather than the mental health trust? Tracy will provide an answer. 'We're in a culture and climate that's busy blaming older people for staying in hospital longer than is needed', she explains, 'and part of my job is to combat that high level of discrimination. This is a big issue'. Tracy may have to defend her patients.

A morning of number-crunching will be followed by an afternoon of stark contrast. Tracy has four new referrals this week. One lady is on an orthopaedic ward, one lady a surgical ward and two gentlemen are on a general medical ward. She will manage to see three patients in person, and have a chat on the phone with the fourth patient's relatives. She is responsible for the admissions and discharges for an eighteen-bedded unit and receives referrals from two large general hospitals and one elderly care site. This is all part of a large caseload: anybody who has dementia on any of these wards could be referred to Tracy.

Between referrals she will take 'phone-calls, and oversee discharge and admission planning. A bed cannot remain empty, but on the other hand no one should be inappropriately placed; patients 'need to have a known diagnosis or chronic confusional problem. We can then do all the medical screening and assessment'. She will probably leave the hospital at 7pm.

Influencing practice

Tracy is routinely 'shadowed' or followed around by trainees – at least once a week. Last week three people shadowed her in one day. Nursing, medical and psychology students, Nurses and service managers are all welcome to watch her work and on Tuesday a third-year medical student – who wants to be a Psychiatrist – will get his turn. Shadowing Tracy will form a key part of his training because he is particularly interested in Lewy Body Dementia, an area about which Tracy is passionate. She explains that people with Lewy Body Dementia are often misdiagnosed and given inappropriate sedative drugs to which they are extremely sensitive,

> 'A lot of the work I do is educational. I need the staff on the ground
> to act as a kind of early warning system to me…if they believe some-
> body might have Lewy Body Dementia I want them to call me.'

The more people Tracy can influence the more effective the service patients receive will become.

09:30–12:30 Tuesday. The head of the Social Work department from the acute hospital needs to update her staff on dementia care and cognitive impairment, so a joint training initiative has been arranged. A Psychiatrist will be talking about 'capacity to consent'. Somebody involved in developing an intermediate care service for people with dementia will also be present. Tracy will run a teaching session about the pros and cons of the Folstein Test. Tracy explains that the Folstein Test – used to make a baseline assessment of cognitive function – is widely misused and misinterpreted. As with Lewy Body Dementia there is a wide gulf between best practice models and clinical reality.

By the time the session is over the social workers should be aware that sweeping generalisations are often made on the back of the Folstein Test and they should be wary of how much it influences their own recommendations. At present many social workers use the Folstein Test as a 'rule of thumb' which Tracy will tell them is 'absolutely not what the test was designed to do'. Again, Tracy is an advocate for patients; she sees a 'big part' of her role to be 'fighting discrimination'.

As a Consultant Nurse Tracy has access to a wide range of people who can prevent discrimination; she has the authority to influence and to persuade, and sharing her expertise is an activity rarely confined to the world of nursing. Of course she advises nurses, and as a consultant she has the authority and expertise to challenge colleagues. She gives an example of a recent generalisation – made by nursing staff – that she challenged. A patient in an orthopaedic setting was labelled as being 'unfit for rehabilitation' because she had dementia. It became clear to Tracy after a brief conversation with the patient in question that she possessed a level of insight that contradicted the 'unfit' description ('these generalisations happen right across disciplines').

Leadership

Tracy is confident that her discussions with the social workers about how they can improve their care plans for people with dementia will be productive and have a wide impact across the service. When the Consultant Nurse role was first suggested there were concerns that it was little more than a 're-badged' nurse specialist role. Tracy, while admitting that she 'doesn't care' if it is or not, believes that the vital difference between the two roles is the leadership element of her job. She knows there are nurse specialists who could become Consultant Nurses. After all, nurse specialists often have 'leadership skills, expertise, are interested in research and training practice development'.

Being a leader means that Tracy has been involved in some very complex and challenging decision-making. But she never sees herself as a 'Super-nurse' making unilateral decisions. Instead she wants to hear what everyone on the team thinks, so she 'pools information together and comes to a mutually agreed position'. In a field historically managed by psychiatry her work in the acute sector is particularly radical. She must be a pioneer. She feels she may have to 'challenge common doctrine, question historical boundaries and empower those who do not believe they have any power' (Packer, 2001).

Research

At 12:30pm on Tuesday Tracy will 'leg-it' to the in-patient unit for people with dementia and meet a final year PhD student. The ward is being used as a pilot site for research into a system that will gather more detailed information about people with dementia, rather than simply reductive facts. In effect the aim is to prevent patients being reduced to 'just a diagnosis'. She admits that the phrase 'person-centred' is a fashionable one at the moment, but that this should not detract from its integrity. Tracy is enthusiastic about the research and wants to see the pilot used and extended widely. It is perhaps a perfect marriage of research and clinical practice and perhaps an indication of how satisfying her role is: she enables the research and the research improves practice.

Tracy is also highly involved in reviewing and evaluating other types of work. She has just finished a review of a valuable research bid, for example, and will offer her opinion on chapters of books (largely to establish suitability for publishing). She is the clinical practice editor of the *Journal of Dementia Care*, and the Department of Health contact her frequently to feed into their work, which she finds particularly exciting.

Opportunities for engagement

2:00pm Tuesday. There will be no time for lunch. Tracy – with shadower in tow-starts the ward round ('the only 'typical' thing about the week'). She will say 'hello' to individuals who have been recently referred, and will chair a multi-disciplinary meeting attended by Physiotherapists, Physiotherapy Assistants, the head of Occupational Therapy, a Social

Worker, the Senior House Officer and Nursing staff. During the meeting the progress of every patient is comprehensively reviewed. There is detailed pain assessment. In her role as a Consultant Nurse she can fundamentally influence the way patients are assessed,

> 'One of the most common difficulties for people with dementia in acute hospitals is they often get accused of being violent and non-compliant when in fact, actually, it *hurts*…they might not have the language and the skills to explain to you, 'look I don't want you to do this to me because it's really hurting me and I can't cope', so they might hit you…it's then perceived that they hit you because they are demented…so we're very big on non-verbal pain assessment. We use the whole team, and the person concerned where possible, to feed into that process.'

This sense of collaboration, and finding radical informed solutions, permeates every aspect of her working life.

The meeting will then go on to look at how the families of the patients are coping and contributing; wherever possible the team like to send people home. Staff problems are discussed ('I'm always challenging the boundaries and the limitations. Let's not look at things as obstacles. Let's find solutions'). The psychosocial interactions of the patients are also examined in detail. This is done to support nursing staff who have developed a model of working which radically involves patients through making use of social interaction, for example in making beds or visiting the Pharmacy. Staff are encouraged to 'see the routines of the day as an opportunity for engagement'.

The ward round finishes at 4:30pm, and the shadower is debriefed. Tracy will then meet three or four sets of relatives. This will mean a late finish on Tuesday but she knows it is crucial to involve families: 'relatives are equal partners in the care process. It's really important for them to feel that they are involved in the decision-making process'. After conversations with relatives she will write up her notes in the medical notes.

It was a hard lesson to learn for Tracy that the four main roles of the Consultant Nurse cannot always be clearly identified on a day-to-day basis. On Tuesday, for example, she will address all of the four main roles of the Consultant Nurse (as set out by the Department of Health) in one day. But she does not make light of being able to do so,

> 'When I was a new Consultant Nurse I really had a sense that I must be able to match my diary against each role. In every report or document that I produce I always use 'those titles' because management understand those boundaries. Those definitions are there to make everybody else feel better. When you're really fluid in your role you don't think, "have I done enough research this week?".'

This sort of fluidity and success has meant that Tracy remains buoyant. She has not become jaded in the role, which in the current NHS climate she finds 'fairly astonishing'. She knows that many of her Consultant Nurse colleagues feel the same: they are saying, 'what a fantastic job'.

New models of care

On Wednesday morning Tracy will meet a clinical psychologist and clinical psychology trainee. She has been working jointly with a renal unit who are interested in older people having dialysis and this collaboration has produced a practical change in the way patients are treated. The team realised there is minimal opportunity for training in renal medicine for staff working with patients who are chronically confused. They also realised that the group of people needing dialysis were as a whole getting older. They squared the circle and developed a working 'model of care'. Practice will be improved and their work will be disseminated in at least three journal articles. This process is about sharing information and expertise across artificial boundaries, a key part of her role. Tracy contributes to curriculum development, nurse training, and post-registration development. University staff see her in an academic context whereas staff on the wards see her in a clinical setting,

> 'It's about leading across boundaries and across professions. You can almost ditch the "nurse". It's not about "nurse" consultancy; it's about being a consultant. As much of my consultancy work is done with social workers, occupational therapists, psychiatrists, doctors, as it is with nurses. My profession is a nurse, and nursing defines my approach, but it doesn't restrict who I am as a consultant.'

Influence on the ward and around the world

At lunchtime on Wednesday Tracy will lead a teaching session with the

Admissions Assessment Unit. This team does not have dementia expertise, and when a confused older person arrives they can get expert information from Tracy:

> 'The minute somebody with dementia enters the service they call me.
> I filter through the people who have delirium but no dementia and
> provide telephone advice and support. I make sure that the people
> with probable dementia are not bounced through five or six wards.'

At the teaching session Tracy will talk about what staff in the assessment unit can do as part of their 'automatic response procedures'. Tracy will suggest certain questions they could ask, or observations they could make, which could speed-up the process of admission. Her advice is evidence-based and because she is constant contact with patients, she does not 'lose touch'.

On Wednesday afternoon Tracy will see referrals. She will also continue to work on the Department of Health report which she began on Monday morning. She wants the report to champion successes; she may choose to include visual materials taken on the ward for the Dementia Service Development training videos. These materials have a large potential audience: 'We're not just any service. We have an impact, not just in the trust that we're in, but we influence knowledge and training around the world'. It is partly up to Tracy to make sure the government gets the whole picture.

Networking and mutual supervisors

At the end of Wednesday afternoon Tracy will meet a fellow Consultant Nurse in the pub. It's midway through the week and they will review and network. She admits that, while it's developing all the time, there is still only a 'fractured' community of Consultant Nurses. And although she receives most of her support from colleagues and peers in the field of dementia care, it is helpful for her to meet other consultants. Over a drink they will be reflective and supportive. They will act as 'mutual supervisors'.

This sharing is a key element of the role:

'This can be a lonely Job. You're in the thick of it a lot of the time and there is still not that many of us around. I have a couple of Consultant Nurse colleagues in the area and we meet up in groups and individually.'

Tracy warns that the job, at times, can be frustrating:

'A lot of the time you're feeling frustrated because you're not doing enough…you go through periods where you think, "I'm not very good at this. I'm not doing all the things everyone wants me to do"…you're often your own worst enemy…'

She believes the annual formal report is an excellent forum in which to evaluate just how much work she has done ('wait a minute, I *have* done a lot this year'). She also has no quibble with the pervasive climate of accountability: 'I don't want us to get in the position where we become like medical consultants have been viewed in the past, where you're beyond scrutiny'. To this end she is in the process of setting up systems to capture the impact of what she is doing, and building 'an evaluative framework' into every aspect of her work.

Drawing the line and stretching the boundaries

With such a huge number of varying commitments it seems incredible that Tracy manages to make room for everything. The fact that she does so is partly due to her skill at saying 'no' gracefully and by acting as a 'signpost' – directing people to other people. When she explains the way she views her responsibilities it becomes clear that she is a master of the balancing act:

'You can be completely overwhelmed by it all…you could go under. One of the hardest lessons I've had to learn is that I can only do what I can do, and as long as I stay true to the fact that I want to work in as person-centred way as possible, and that patients come first…I suspect that that is a dilemma that faces all Consultant Nurses: where you draw the line.'

On Thursday morning Tracy will conduct interviews for her new secretary. The fact that she didn't have one for three years was a problem,

'The kind of systems I'd have liked to have been in place haven't been...I need someone who can cope with the relatives' calls...I receive international enquiries...there are distraught relatives...this person isn't just a secretary, they're a lynchpin that could make or break the service.'

Thursday afternoon is a time to talk to any relatives who Tracy didn't manage to see on Tuesday. She will make a range of 'phone-calls, mainly about service development within the Trust; there are a number of groups involved in strategic service development, including two other Consultant Nurses (one involved in GPs' surgeries and one in community interventions) who work collaboratively, in part to ensure that work is not being replicated inappropriately.

Tracy works very closely with a Professor of Medicine. Together they are devising 'treatment diagnostic protocols' to enable Tracy to formally diagnose and treat urine infections, urinary retention and constipation,

'I'm taking on diagnostic and treatment stuff which is usually what doctors do. As a Consultant Nurse part of what I do is stretch the boundaries of what's happening. So by learning some diagnostic interventions our patients can get treated sooner and more effectively without hanging around waiting for doctors to sign a form.'

She has an excellent relationship with the Professor, who provides support and is receptive. She now has full admission, discharge and referral rights ('For some Consultant Nurses it's been a real battle just to get that, so that feels good'). She has not experienced the reported lack of role-credibility or lack of support from medics,

'Doctors make referrals to me. I make referrals to doctors. I've been involved in medical student training. I've worked alongside consultants training. I make referrals to psychiatrists...if anything it was harder for the nursing staff to get their head around what I was about.'

The Professor of Medicine handed over large parts of his former role to Tracy because he realised it was 'logical'. The fluidity and novelty of her role means that it always adapting, mutating and evolving.

Teaching and mentoring

On Friday morning Tracy is teaching in the Occupational Health department ('I love that I teach so many different groups of people'). They request a session from her once every three months and it makes a real difference to working practices. At the last session Tracy talked to the entire department about what dementia is and is not: 'it's made a real difference to what they were doing'. She will discuss some of the legal and ethical issues surrounding dementia, including consent and decision-making for discharge planning. She will refer to the Human Rights Act and some case law that has been effective over the past couple of years. Crucially, she will field questions and try to apply theory to everyday situations.

Later on Tracy meets a ward manager she is mentoring. She meets with her for an hour a month at midday on Fridays. The Ward Manager wants to become a Consultant Nurse in transitional care. Then Tracy will have a meeting with the Director of Nursing for the Primary Care Trust during which they will talk about the development of dementia services in the coming years.

No neat answers

In between the meetings, mentoring, and teaching Tracy will pick up more referrals and make 'phone calls to relatives. People call from around the country. A typical enquiry may be from a ward that is keeping people with dementia in a side-room at night because they are 'being disruptive'. They ask Tracy's opinion. She will want to know if the patients are having something to eat and drink before bed, if they are craving the social contact of the night staff, or perhaps going to the toilet and getting lost. She will explain that there are no neat answers.

Tracy will have a day off on Saturday and run a carers support group on Sunday. Carers will share information, offer support, receive support, and work through feelings. The meetings can be fun, but there is much anger, sadness and pain. The week will present emotional as well as intellectual challenges.

The real story of real people

Tracy sees her ability to come off the clinical floor and influence service development at the strategic level as a key part of her role,

> 'A Consultant Nurse works across the boundaries. It's not just about nursing…how will my leadership skills mean that I can go into a Trust Board meeting and make a case for why a service should be developed in a particular way? The reason I can is because that morning I was with this patient or this family and this was their experience…the real story of real people.'

But Tracy is as deluged by conference requests as she is with calls from anxious relatives. She feels comfortable doing a job with such a range of responsibilities: 'I'm in a job that I love, with status and credibility and a respectable salary. A sizeable chunk of my time is spent making a difference clinically. What more do I want?'

She has, potentially, another thirty years in the NHS. She does not want to be a Consultant Nurse for all of them. What's next? The consultant role has raised her expectations:

> 'When I was a junior nurse I aspired to be a Ward Manager. When I became a Ward Manager I aspired to be a specialist nurse and then didn't know what to do, then aspired to be a Consultant Nurse. I'm now a Consultant Nurse. What do I aspire to be? I aspire to be a Clinical Chair and that's what I think will happen. Part of my role now is making people think about the need for that role in the future.'

The role has given her opportunities she would never have had otherwise: travel to Australia, the USA and Europe, teaching and networking.

When she speaks her audiences will not just hear about dementia care, they will hear how she is inventing her role.

References

Packer, T (2001) Acute Care Series Part 1: a consultant nurse in dementia care. *Signpost* 5(3), February, p. 20.

CHAPTER THREE

Ordinary expertise

Gary Wilshaw & Geoff Speight

Introduction

In this chapter, we reflect on the nature of 'expertise' in the context of mental health nursing and the role of the Consultant Nurse. Health Service Circular 1999/217 refers to the 'expert practice' element of the Consultant Nurse role, but does not develop the idea much beyond the expectation that the post-holder will hold a higher degree. It could be argued that this requirement alone is relatively meaningless, and fails to help us understand what exemplary nursing practice actually looks like.

We intend to use the opportunity of this chapter to share ideas on the nature of expertise in this context. From the outset we should state that we are motivated by a deep concern that current wisdom is developing in a way that sees nursing as a merely technical, 'nursing-by-numbers' process. Many well-motivated nurses appear to be convinced that the application of 'manual' based formulaic treatments offers a model of what is best-practice in nursing, and by implication, a model of 'expertise' that might be witnessed in the Consultant Nurse. What works is crucial to purposeful activity in nursing, and therefore need to be embraced. However, these ideas are not the *totality* of nursing. Instead, we believe that they are facets of a basis for practice to be considered as *data*, and as with all data, there is a need for further analysis, context setting and interpretation.

'Extended roles' in nursing

In some areas of nursing, roles have been 'extended' to incorporate 'new' functions such as nurse-prescribing; cannulation & venepuncture (Levenson & Vaughan, 1999). Castledine (1998) points out that much of this 'development' either mirrors medical traditions in the division of labour, or reflects a model of the medical 'treatment' of a 'condition' (such as cancer), and applies the same thinking to so-called 'conditions' of the mind. This piecemeal approach to role development has characterised developments in nursing, especially 'adult' (general) nursing, for some time and seems to be evidence for a deep-seated fondness for – and affiliation with – the medical model and the work of doctors. Some mental health nurses are, of course, aware and critical of this bogus 'development' process. Speight (2003) reported his incredulity at the energy some of his senior mental health nursing colleagues were putting into developing the agenda of 'nurse-prescribing'. His exasperated question to his colleagues was simply 'why would you want to prescribe drugs?'

> Imagine the following scenario: I'm with a group of mental health nurses at a seminar, and the introductions run as follows; 'Hi, I'm John and I use Psycho-social and early interventions with patients', 'Hi, I'm a cognitive behavioural therapist and can help patients to change their negative schemas', 'Hi, I'm a supplementary prescriber and can alter the dose of medication for my patients, What about yourself?' '... well, I said with some trepidation, I'm Geoff ... and I just try to understand, listen to, and care for my patients, who are often struggling with experiences they can't understand'
> The rest of the group denounced this as 'lacking focus, lacking an evidence base and low grade work best left to support workers'.
>
> (Speight, 2003, personal communication)

If Consultant Nurses are to lead innovation and development in healthcare, it is not enough to simply take part in the redistribution of work already being done by others – for example, doctors. The best that could be hoped for from this approach is the maintenance of the status quo.

We find it sad to note the extent to which nursing embarrassed itself during the final decades of the 20th century, with talk of a range of 'levels of competence' of its members (UKCC, 1992, 1994, 1997). Conference speakers and learned journal paper writers have urged nurses to seriously discriminate the finer points of nursing practice, and this is reflected in job titles such as Clinical Nurse Specialist, Advanced Practitioner, Nurse Practitioner, Senior Clinical Nurse, Specialist Nurse Practitioner and others. Our point here is not to criticise this work per se, but to point out the serious risk of incoherence and of taking our eye off the ball. For the Consultant Nurse to represent anything different than is offered by this unseemly scramble to coin an impressive job title, a coherent and mature understanding of the nature of clinical expertise, and a means of exploiting this, is needed. Not for the first time mental health nursing has an opportunity to break the mould being cast for us all, and to re-examine the notion of expertise and the role of the nurse.

Conscience and humanity in nursing

In some areas of mental health care, the fondness for the medical model has been less intense. Nurses, Occupational Therapists and Social Workers are leading innovations and developments in ways that are less dependent upon the technical, often mainly pharmaceutical skills, of the doctor. Perhaps it is pertinent here to reflect on our history and heritage.

Charles Mercier, a pioneering alienist, in his instructions to attendants for the insane wrote *"The first duty of an attendant, then is to treat his patients with kindness, gentleness and humanity, both in deed and in word"* (Mercier, 1898 p3). We would submit that to lose sight of the humanity and experience of the patient, amidst the technical expertise of the professional, is to fall at the first hurdle. For a useful review of ideas related to the emergence of the modern mental health nurse from these beginnings the reader is referred to Nolan (1990).

In mental health nursing, the work of Peplau (e.g. 1986), Barker (1997a, 1997b), Barker, Reynolds & Stevenson (1997) and others, has been instrumental in the development and sustenance of an essential *humanity* in the practise of mental health nursing. This has helped mental health nursing develop a sense of *conscience*, and in turn avoid the wholesale reduction of the personal and individual *meaning* of mental suffering to mere components of professional activity. This humane approach has much in common with the Moral Treatment system of care pioneered by William Tuke and the Quakers at The Retreat in York. This was an attempt to create an environment which provided humane care in a homely setting, for people who were 'afflicted' by the loss of reason. It also added the concept of treating the mentally ill as though they were mentally *well*.

Tuke (1813) essentially managed a lay experiment in caring for the mentally unwell, with physicians playing a peripheral role. The Retreat embodied the principles of a therapeutic community, with staff and patients living, eating and working together. Medical treatments were offered, but it would appear that more often than not they failed to produce tangible benefits. Staff would then abandon those methods and rely instead on an ordinary wisdom, a commonsense approach and intuition.

Such an approach today would of course, evoke derision and would be abandoned as a result of its inability to provide sufficient positivistic data. Scull (1989) expresses a key mismatch of the approach to contemporary fashion – that is – its rejection of any central notion of 'expert or specialist skills', means that it is not supportive of a narrative that is about enhancing professional power. The essential component of moral treatment was its emphasis on humanity, and such a quality, Tuke felt, is not one that should be monopolized by experts. This perhaps illustrates the dynamics at play when people are developing decent and helpful approaches to those who are suffering. On the one hand there is the imperative to do what is *right*, and on the other hand there is the agenda of serving political and professional interests. These two paths are not mutually exclusive – but difficult and mature choices may have to made from time to time.

An opportunity exists for the Consultant Nurse at this time of optimism about the new role to make the right choice. Incumbents have it in their gift to avoid fragmentation and reduction of the job into disparate and discrete components. By doing so a contribution can be made to the effort to avoid reduction, dismissal and objectification of the individual experience of suffering.

The nature of expert practice for the Consultant Nurse

The Consultant Nurse in mental health must model excellence in care delivery – but let us think for a moment what this means. To us, excellent practice refers to conduct that is characterised, perhaps paradoxically, by a modest deference to the wisdom gained through the experience of mental suffering. By taking a lead from the person experiencing mental distress, the Consultant Nurse recognises singularity of experience and resists the pressure to apply 'textbook wisdom'.

Whether or not the relationship between the patient and the Consultant Nurse is to be significant or insignificant may be determined, argues McQueen (2000), by the primacy given to what he calls 'presencing'. This refers to a responsive 'being-with' the patient (Benner & Wrubel, 1989) in both an emotional and physical sense. It is not difficult to think of this relational quality as a well-developed empathy that goes well-beyond the mere attendance to the patient and their problems.

Mearns & Thorne (2000) rather apologetically preface their re-visiting of the concept of Carl Rogers' 'core conditions', with a heart-felt justification that is relevant to the discussion here. They point out that many counsellors, therapists and others (and by implication – nurses) have developed a *rhetorical habit* of speaking of the importance of the relationship between the helper and the patient. In our experience, this throwaway comment has been adopted by many as a foil, designed to subtly denounce the value of out-of-fashion human intimacy and nurturing-based approaches.

The late Annie Altschul (1972) was one such advocate of this seemingly unfashionable approach. She was passionately committed to the notion that an interpersonal relationship with patients was the core of mental health nursing. The current demands placed on mental health nurses and the drive to adopt increasingly 'evidenced' and/or time-limited interventions seriously threatens such an approach. The Draft Mental Health Bill (DoH 2002) is one example among many policies, which is likely to further discount such ideals. Indeed some commentators forecast an ever-increasing push for mental health nurses to abandon the focus on therapeutic relationships and adopt an increasingly 'policing type role' to placate growing public anxiety (Morrall, 1998; Speight, 1994). Perhaps we need to be wary of recent innovations, technologies and policies that potentially threaten the ideals of essential mental health nursing practice.

To pick up again on the point that Mearns and Thorne (2000) raise, many senior mental health nurses now mechanically suggest that *of course*, application of the pre-designed technique is always preceded by the development of a 'good relationship'. Thus the relationship is seen as forming merely a basis from which to apply further instrumental technique – in other words, a power-base is aimed at from which to exert leverage. What is revealed in this mechanism is a misunderstanding of the place of those very intimate dimensions of connectedness (Dyson, 1997) in the process of healing. Mearns & Thorne (2000) point out that these dimensions are not mere mechanical prerequisites, to be put into place before the mechanics of repair can then be executed. Instead they point to a weight of evidence in support of an intrinsic healing quality in the experience of being valued and closely understood within a caring relationship – processes that we feel are at the heart of mental health nursing, and that are currently under threat. These ideas are echoed in the more contemporary ideas of Clarkson (1994) and Friedman (1995) who speak respectively of the replenishing potential of the therapeutic relationship where there may be developmentally rooted deficits impeding the well-being of the individual. The late David Brandon (1997), who himself had experience of been on the receiving end of mental health services, was deeply suspicious of therapy. He makes a plea for relationships between 'user' and professional, to be less 'professional' and much more 'everyday' (the sort of relationship in which a deep and mutual respect for each other might flourish).

There needs to be an appreciation of the value of intuition. An expert practitioner should be one who can use both their knowledge of effective interventions and their experience of different situations, to intuitively chart a course of action which is right for that patient.

Consultant Nursing and spirituality

The Hebrew word for spirit – 'ruah' – translates as 'wind' or 'breath'. It is interesting to note that the 'inspired' person may be enlivened, vigorous or 'spirited', and that we may speak of the depressed person as 'dispirited on uninspired. The hint we are given, in this derivational diversion, is that there is a role for the Consultant Nurse to embrace the spiritual dimension of nursing, and a chance to offer a lead or *validation* of this concept to others.

Spirituality is sometimes associated with the finding of *meaning* in life (Goldberg, 1998), or finding a purpose to live (Martsolf, 1998) when direction is lost or suffering so overwhelming that one's coping resources are inadequate. An implication is that the therapeutic relationship may be a place to begin to search for such meaning and explanations of what is felt to be significant in life. Indeed for at least a while, the relationship may *be* the object of meaning for some. Often, to succeed is to become inspired or to regain one's spirit, and to achieve this a depth of connect-edness (Dyson, 1997) between the nurse and the patient is needed *or* the connectedness itself may provide the sense of meaning.

Any nurse claiming to be an expert then, needs to be comfortable with an experience described by Clarkson (1994) as being jointly – if tem-porarily – 'lost' alongside the patient, both with a deep sense of appreci-ation of each other at an essentially personal or spiritual level. The challenge of course, is for the 'expert' nurse to manage such an experience within therapeutic boundaries that permit subsequent development and perhaps a sense of learning and hope. This aspect of caring and being cared for is potentially an aspect of love. We need to guard against self-satisfying motives (*epithymia* and *eros*) but not let that detract from mov-ing toward identification with others (fellow-feeling, *philia*) and maybe even further still, where there is genuine concern for the welfare of others (value-enhancing love *agape,* Lewis 1960). It is well summed by Williams (1968, p.3): 'Love means a willingness to participate in the being of the other at the cost of suffering, and with the expectation of mutual enrich-ment, criticism and growth.'

A circle of friends

In North East Yorkshire, Scarborough MIND has developed a concept they have named the 'Circle of Friends'. The model is one in which peo-ple are put in touch with 'friends' that are willing to 'supply' from a range of five key functions which are:

1. Emotional support (including a 'listening ear')
2. Practical support (including help with shopping or with childcare)
3. Information (including reliable material on helping agencies)
4. Advocacy (including speaking up for someone when they would value this)
5. Social support (including assistance to the isolated).

The model appears to be successful (it is currently being evaluated) and has offered well-evaluated assistance to around one hundred local people at the time writing. The reason we include mention of this work here, is that the unifying model that underlies the work is *friendship*. The impact that is being reported does not just concern the delivery of the initial task agreed with the person by the volunteer, but also includes an additional sense of *community and belonging* that begins to develop after the initial tasks are complete.

The friendship model lacks the pretence of 'special skill' or expertise, and instead, modestly places its value in its ordinariness and sense of the everyday.

The stupid expert

In contrast to the thinking within 'Circle of Friends', Brandon (2000) suggests how a person (e.g. a nurse) may become 'stupid' by being 'chronically self righteous' or dogmatic – by knowing what is 'best' in the care of others. Rowe (1989) even suggests such people are dangerous and should be avoided by those feeling in need of emotional help. For the 'expert' Consultant Nurse to avoid being dangerous or 'stupid' in this sense, they might well be advised to experiment with what Brandon (2000) describes as a 'beginners mind'.

Here, a freshness of being is taken to his or her encounters with the person in care, which leaves him or her truly receptive to that individual's way of experiencing suffering. The Consultant Nurse need not aspire to heroism, compelled to demonstrate superior knowledge and skills that may amount to no more than ego-enhancing rescue attempts. Indeed we would argue that the current push to develop specialist therapeutic skills, has partly succeeded in focussing the concerns of mental health nurses more on themselves and these interventions. In the process nurses have become less concerned with the experience of the person in receipt of these skills. The essence of nursing – the nurturing of others – does not need such machismo, but instead, perhaps *demands* a gentleness and wisdom that may cultivate communication networks and a nourishing climate. It is interesting to note that we do not believe seeking therapeutic skill is *in itself* dangerous in its potential to distract from the person in care and their needs. Rather, it is a reminder that to handle or *integrate* such new skills into one's essential humanity, is not an easy task that all will to do with ease.

The adoption of Brandon's (2000) freshness may require a greater strength and maturity than is at first obvious. It may be that the

Consultant Nurse is very well placed to model such a posture in the same sense that a truly effective leader does not need to thump their chest and browbeat others into the acceptance of their ideas. Having achieved the most senior clinical position available, the Consultant Nurse has an opportunity to listen and to understand, to embrace ideas, to build consensus among colleagues and support others – in short, the need to impress others has gone.

This state of mind is not the same as ignorance. The expert Consultant Nurse is not disabled by an openness to the wisdom of experience, they will simply embrace it and allow it to be their principal guide. Similarly, the jointly 'lost' experience (Clarkson, 1994) with the patient described above, is a temporary experience of mutuality with the patient. Alongside this, there is plenty of opportunity for the Consultant Nurse to be extremely well informed, educated and analytically minded, to have well-developed research skills and be an inspirational leader. Indeed there is a certain *potency* suggested when the well-prepared (in an educational/training/experience sense) nurse is able to reveal a measured but genuine uncertainty or bewilderment, alongside the patient, and with colleagues.

A willingness to avoid the use of qualifications and training as a *defence*, and therefore to *block* any encounter of two persons in the 'I-Thou' sense (Buber, 1970) is required of this expert Consultant Nurse. The healing potential of such an encounter is well argued by Buber (1970) and others (e.g. Woskett, 1999, Campbell 1984) and is concerned with the sharing of an essential humanity rather than the deployment of discrete technical skills. As we see it, the real skill required of this 'expert' is to retain something of the ordinariness one should bring as a human being, whilst simultaneously developing perfectly valid skills concerning the 'therapeutic use of self' (e.g. Peplau, 1986; Butterworth, 1987; Woskett, 1999), use of transference, core belief restructuring or sophisticated family work skills based on systems theory, for example.

Organisational level expertise

In addition to the modelling of expertise when working with individual patients or families, the Consultant Nurse must win a comparable stature in the relevant organisation. Mirroring the sentiments of these reflections so far, this is achieved perhaps paradoxically, via a suspension of pretensions to know what is best.

Instead, our belief is that expertise at this level is founded upon sensitivity to the needs of individuals, teams, communities and the organisations that make up the whole system of care. It is characterised by the seeking of alliances with agencies within the whole system, comparable to therapeutic alliances found in the most effective care relationships (Lidz & Lidz, 1994; Wade, 1995; Miller *et al.*, 1997).

In setting out to work in this way, there are clearly a number of great challenges. One such challenge is that, currently, Consultant Nurse posts do not contain line management or executive 'power' over key staff. A further challenge is that the Consultant Nurse cannot *lead* by merely 'tuning in' to the locality and offering support to dynamics already at play. The leadership role demands a vision and strength of character to follow an idea through, including when there is resistance. Just as the expert nurse may 'challenge' the patient within the context of a sound therapeutic relationship, so they must challenge the *organisation*, or its components, to address it's denial, self-deceit, game-playing or lethargy. The Consultant Nurse must also be able to offer alternatives to these unhelpful strategies and be able to model these in everyday encounters.

To fulfil these complex tasks the Consultant Nurse needs to be in day-to-day close working relationships with those that manage and set the strategic direction, and also those that 'deliver the goods' in the caring settings. This places a great strain on the incumbent, as there is difficult boundary maintenance work to be done. On the one hand the Consultant is working shoulder-to-shoulder with clinicians and patients on matters of direct care, and in doing this is experiencing first-hand the realities of working for this particular organisation. On the other hand they are influencing strategic direction and sharing in the work of management at the most senior level. In doing so, the Consultant Nurse may be seen as a *part* of the senior management structure, making the development of a substantive *trust* with fellow clinical workers more of a challenge if there are issues of mistrust in place. As explored elsewhere in this book, the fact that the Consultant Nurse connects to so many aspects of the work of the local system of healthcare may be an enormous strength, adding as it does a certain credibility and awareness of 'real', day-to-day clinical issues.

Discussion and conclusions

For systems of care to be coherent, the underlying philosophy, beliefs and values must be reflected in everyday practice. A lack of coherence will be 'visible' in that what is espoused as a value does not match the experience of the majority of users of those services.

We believe there is still a narrative of elitism in nursing and healthcare, and that this will sabotage aspirations to build user-led systems and develop care that is truly valuable and valued. Part of this elitism remains rooted in the re-emergence of positivism and modernism. These forces support empiricism and 'objectivity' at all costs, and denounce that which is considered 'subjective'. The drive for increased professional status will undoubtedly create further elitism. Professions by their nature lay claim to and guard their knowledge. This is exemplified in the current pre and post-registration nurse training, therapy training and personal development that devalues the personal and direct experience of students, serves to support elitism and dis-articulation from the experience of suffering. Elitism suggests that professionals know best, and that the greater the salary or grander the job title the more this is true. Consultant Nurses have a unique opportunity to buck this trend and offer a model of expertise that is non-elitist.

The fundamental role of the nurse, hinted at in the derivation of the verb to 'nurse', is to provide an environment in which the person in need may be *nourished*. For the Consultant Nurse, it is not enough to do this in a direct and one-to-one sense alone. The opportunity on offer for the incumbent is to influence the whole system and health care community to move towards a *culture* of nourishment, where a depth of relationship between service users, carers and paid staff is fostered and valued. This culture is not characterised by a glittering array of technical skill deployment, but instead is revealed in its valuing of emotional contact, and sense of friendship and attachment.

References

Altschul A. (1972) *Patient-nurse interaction: A study of interaction patterns in acute psychiatric wards.* Churchill Livingstone, Edinburgh.

Barker P. (1997a) The craft of care, collaborative caring in psychiatric nursing. In: Tilley S (ed.) *The mental health nurse.* Routledge, London.

Barker P. (1997b) Towards a meta-theory of psychiatric nursing practice. *Mental Health Practice* 1(4) 18–21.

Barker P. Reynolds C., Stevenson C. (1997) The human science basis of psychiatric nursing *Journal of Advanced Nursing*, 25, 660–667.

Benner P. Wrubel J. (1989) *The primacy of caring*. Addison-Wesley, London.

Brandon D. (1997) *The trick of being ordinary*. Anglia Polytechnic University, Cambridge.

Brandon D. (2000) *The tao of survival*. Venture Press, Birmingham.

Buber M. (1970) *I and Thou* (Kaufmann translation) T & T Clarke, Edinburgh.

Butterworth T. (1987) Psychiatric nursing: fumbling in a vacuum or grasping an opportunity *Mental Health Nursing: the Journal of the Psychiatric Nurses Association October*, 6.

Campbell A.V. (1984) *Moderated love: A theology of professional care*. SPCK. London.

Castledine G. & McGee P. (eds) (1998) *Advanced and specialist nursing practice*. Routledge, London.

Clarkson P. (1994) The psychotherapeutic relationship. In: Clarkson P & Pokorny M (eds) *The handbook of psychotherapy*. Routledge, London.

Friedman M. (1995) *The healing dialogue in psychotherapy*. Jason-Aranson, New York.

Goldberg B. (1998) Connection: an exploration of spirituality in nursing care *Journal of Advanced Nursing*, 27(4) pp. 836–842.

Levenson R. & Vaughan B. (1999) *Developing new roles in practice: an evidence-based guide*. SCHARR, University of Sheffield, Sheffield.

Lewis C.S. (1960) *The four loves*. Collins. Glasgow.

Lidz T., Lidz R.W. (1994) Curative factors in the psychotherapy of schizophrenic patients. In Slipp S (ed.) *Curative factors in dynamic psychotherapy*. McGraw-Hill, London.

Martsolf D. (1998) The concept of spirituality in nursing theories: differing world views and extent of focus *Journal of Advanced Nursing*, 27(2) pp. 294–303.

Mearns D., Thorne B. (2000) *Person centred therapy today*. Sage, London.

Mercier C., (1898) *The Attendant's Companion*. 2nd ed. J&A Churchill London.

Miller S.D., Duncan B.L., Hubble M.A. (1997) *Escape from Babel: towards a unifying language for psychotherapy practice*. Norton, New York.

McQueen A. (2000) Nurse–patient relationships and partnerships in hospital care *Journal of Clinical Nursing*, 9(5) pp 723–731.

Morrall P. (1998) *Mental Health Nursing and Social Control*. Whurr Publishers London.

Nolan P. (1990) Psychiatric nursing – the first hundred years *Journal of Advanced Nursing*, 18, 44–47.

Peplau H. (1986) Hildegard Peplau: Grand Dame of psychiatric nursing (interview) *Geriatric Nursing*, 7(6), 328–330.

Rowe D. (1989) In: *Against Therapy*. Mason, J Collins, London.

Scull A.T. (1989) *Social Order/Mental Disorder: Anglo-American Psychiatry in Historical Perspective*. University of California Press, Berkeley.

Speight G.K. (1994) *From custody to care? An examination of the passage of the mentally ill from institution to community*. Unpublished MA Thesis University of Central Lancashire.

Tuke S. (1813) *Description of the Retreat, An Institution Near York for Insane Persons of the Society of Friends*. Reprinted by Policy Press 1996.

UKCC (1992) *The scope of professional practice*. UKCC, London.

UKCC (1992) *The future of professional practice. The council's standards for education and practice following registration* UKCC, London.

UKCC (1992) *Specialist practice: considerations of issues relating to embracing nurse practitioners and clinical nurse specialists within the specialist practice framework*. UKCC, London.

Wade S. (1995) Partnership in care: a critical review *Nursing Standard* 9(48) pp 29–32.

Williams D.D. (1968) *The spirit and the forms of love*. Nisbett, London.

Woskett V. (1999) *The therapeutic use of self*. Routledge, London.

CHAPTER FOUR

Who cares anymore, anyway?

Phil Barker

Reclaiming the story of madness

The history of psychiatry is little over one hundred years old but the history of madness extends from the Ancient World to today's so-called 'mental health' system and its associated movements. The ancient Greeks' appreciation of melancholy, differed little from contemporary 'scientific' accounts (Barker, 1992), and the establishment of the first 'asylums' by monks in Northumbria, almost one thousand years ago, find an echo in the contemporary development of 'crisis houses' (Barker, 2002). Although much has been made of the potential of neuroscience to resolve the problems of living that commonly are called 'mental illnesses' (Szasz, 1996), many of the contemporary developments in mental health appear to be trying to re-connect with the emancipatory values of Tuke and Pinel. *Plus ça change?*

Whereas psychiatric medicine has come to focus on the mind as brain, mental distress may be a more complex human phenomenon. Szasz (1996) noted tellingly that:

> 'The material substrates of a human being – a person – are organs, tissues, cells, molecules, atoms, and subatomic particles. The material substrates of a human artifact – say a wedding ring – are crystals, atoms, electrons in orbits, and so forth. Scientists do not claim to be able to explain the economic or emotional value of a wedding ring by identifying its material composition; nor do they insist that a physicalist account of its structure is superior to a cultural and personal account of its meaning.' (p. 140)

Without doubt 'we' express something of who 'we' are, through the biological machinery of brain/mind. It could not be otherwise. However, who 'we' are, is not to be found *in* the brain, in the same way that the television actors, their world of experience and the myriad characters who conspire to produce the play, are not to be found by taking the back off the television set. The *state* of being human is a social phenomenon – defined broadly by the history of civilisations and more locally by influence of culture. The *experience* of being human is a deeply personal phenomenon. Many who reflect on their sense of place in the world fear that their unique vision means that they face the fickleness of Fate alone. Whether or not this is illusory counts for naught. The dark experience of isolation, commonly associated with most forms of so-called mental illness, is often the most significant dividend returned by the art of introspection. The French poet, Gerard de Nerval wrote:

> 'I am the darkly shaded, the bereaved, the inconsolate, the prince of Aquitaine, with the blasted tower. My only star is dead, and my starstrewn lute carries on it the black sun of melancholy.'

Madness is no more or less than story – part social discourse, part personal construction. We each try to build our lives – or at least make sense of the architecture of the self – against the backdrop of socio-cultural values concerning what it means to be human, and the conflicting sense of what it means to be 'me' (Barker, 2003).

For those who try to help people in states of madness the challenge involves entering someone else's story, without entirely losing contact with one's own story; and without imposing the lessons learned in one's own story, on the other.

We are the stories of our lives – no more and no less. This philosophical building block needs to be laid, otherwise nothing else said in this chapter, the name of compassionate caring, will make much sense.

The experience of madness involves a breakdown of understanding or relatedness. The person often feels obliged to retreat from the world of ordinary relationships with others, or their interpersonal discourse becomes highly problematic. People often become acutely self-aware, and experience an emotional terrorism, within which they appear to haunt themselves or at least dog their own experiential footsteps. Given this context, it is hardly surprising that the concept of *recovery* has gained such a powerful presence in the field of what once was known as psychiatric rehabilitation. The person who loses control over life, through the process of mental distress, needs to recover control – reclaiming the life that has been submerged by mental distress. Arguably, the recovery process involves reclaiming the story of madness, as a first step to acknowledging the central position of the story of recovery and reclamation in all our lives.

Caring as a therapeutic modality

Caring was once a simple, lowly process, involving mainly human contact and relations with patients,[1] and their families. The lowly practice of nursing was reinforced, theoretically, by Virginia Henderson's definition of the supportive practice of caring. In the ICNs *Basic Principles of Nursing Care* (Henderson, 1969) she emphasised that 'the physician is regarded as pre-eminent in diagnosis, prognosis and therapy'. However, by the early 1970s several theories of nursing had already been established, which emphasised the therapeutic function of the *caring* concept. Most had strong bases in humanism and holism – especially Travelbee's therapeutic use of self, Watson's science of human caring, and Leininger's transcultural nursing. All placed caring at the heart of nursing, arguably defining this as the *essence* of nursing (Barker *et al.*, 1995; Peck, 1992; Sourial, 1997).

The importance of caring, irrespective of who offers it, has become clearer over the past two decades. Practitioners have developed their awareness that caring *for* someone is quite different from simply caring *about* the person, and the recent emphasis on emancipatory systems has revealed a third dimension – caring *with* the patient (Barker and Whitehill, 1997).

In nursing, caring has been projected more as an attitude than an action, although without the action, the attitude becomes mere rhetoric (Barker, 2000). 'Courage' may not hold a high profile in the public image of nursing, but many nurses attest to its importance in many diverse situations (Brvzczynska, 1997; Fowler, 1996; Lanara, 1981). By adopting an existential ethic, many caring theorists emphasised the dynamic nature of the decision-making in nursing practice (Burnard, 1997; Parse, 1981;

---

[1] I use the term *patients* here partly for ease of expression, partly to avoid the political correctness of the user/consumer/survivor discourse, and partly in recognition of the obvious fact that people do need to be very patient, as they wait for something appropriate to be done to help them in their moment of distress.

Watson, 1988). Some nursing theorists, like Benner and Wrubel (1989), emphasised the power of existential philosophy for nurses, which derives from Heidegger's influence (1962), although he said little about human relationships (Bradshaw, 1996), but shared with Buddhism and Taoism the appreciation that *being* and the universal world spirit were one and the same. That kind of existential ethic – where compassion for fellow humans and any living thing need not differ – stands in sharp contrast to the relationality of Buber (1970) or Frankl's (1964) search for meaning in the face of suffering or death. Such philosophies – more representative of the Judaeo Christian ethic of compassion (and caring) – underpin the theoretical writings of the lay Carmelite, Travelbee (1971) and Patterson and Zderad (1976).

Within most of the nursing theory influenced by existentialism, people are perceived as being in a constant state of flux, engaged in an ongoing process of becoming (Barker, 2001). This applies to people as nurses, as well as to people as patients. Some theorists located this flux of becoming at the heart of their theorising (e.g. Parse, 1981). Under such conditions, caring becomes something of an act of faith (Burnard, 1997), with obvious implications for the issue of 'evidence-based practice'.

The complexity of relating to patients was articulated by Peplau (1952) and later by Travelbee (1971) – who coined the phrase, the *therapeutic use of self*. This suggested the potential of whatever might be going on between nurses and their patients – if not the invisible skill of healing, then the largely invisible ordering of the conditions that might allow healing to take place. This paved the way for the discrimination of more discrete factors involved in caring (Watson, 1988) highlighting the potential importance of even more abstract interpersonal processes, like *vigilance* (Carr, 1998) or *presence* (Owen-Mills, 1998). These developments retained the humanistic–existential frame of reference, and emphasised the dynamic mutuality of the nurse–patient relationship.

More recently, various alternative practices have been woven through the caring attitude. From the complementary medicine perspective, caring is just one process in the nurse's toolbox, which now includes such diverse processes as drawing, acupressure, guided imagery, storytelling, therapeutic touch, soft music and humour (Ward, 1998). Whether these actually *heal* or merely provide the conditions under which healing might take place remains unclear and may not be all that important.

Despite the attractiveness of the caring method the wrapping may be more important than the contents. Bradshaw (1994, 1997) advocated strongly for the primacy of the humanity and personhood inherent in the caring ethic, which she saw threaded through the Judaeo-Christian tradition (*cf* Travelbee, 1971; Paterson and Zderad, 1976). Contemporary developments amplify our appreciation of caring practices. For example, Kempe's (1994) attempts to discriminate different dimensions of presence, as alliances between the nurse and the family caregiver are formed in the emergency care context. Other researchers have explored the possibilities of incorporating existing theories of caring within new models, which emphasises a synthesis of nursing and medical care. Dunphy and Winland-Browns (1998) 'Circle of Caring', for example, highlighted the nursing voice in a rapidly changing healthcare system. Caring is, however, more than just a professional emotional response to distress. Caring generates power within relationships, and, when used appropriately, can help patients (and arguably nurses) to evolve as persons. Where used differently, it may engender dependency. The fact that 'caring' can (and often does) generate negative outcomes, suggests the need for a reflexive definition:

> Caring occurs when growth, healing or recovery occurs
>
> (e.g. Cora, 1998)

> When dependency or harm develops, some other human process is at work
>
> (e.g. Holden, 1991)

Much of the caring literature is North American. However, some theories, such as Watson's science of human caring, appear to cross social and cultural borders (Martin, 1997) and are compatible with multiculturalism (Eddins and Riley-Eddins, 1997). Studies of patient's perceptions of important caring qualities in other cultures – e.g. Muslim societies – bear a remarkable similarity to those in the Western literature (e.g. Nahas, 1997). However, there remains a need to clarify (Dyson, 1997: Gaut, 1993: Greenhalgh *et al.*, 1998) and analyse further the concept (McCance *et al.*, 1997). Some important steps in this direction have been taken in distinguishing the functions of compassion, empathy and altruism, as dimensions of caring, and others have tried to study empirically the effects of formal education on knowledge of, and attitudes towards caring, as well as patterns of caring behaviour themselves (Yang and Lu, 1998).

The development of business-based health care systems may have stimulated an increased demand for caring (Barker *et al.*, 1999; Duffield and Limby, 1994). Although caring is central to the patient's determinant of quality, it incurs little obvious cost. Its invisibility, in economic terms, suggests the need for further clarification of the concept, not only in theoretical function, but also in measuring its effect, in economic terms. That dimension might well be the critical route to preserving caring as part of future healthcare systems, and might be the spur nursing needs to develop an evidence-base that reflects the true importance of caring.

A page from Sue's story[2]

I believe my 'breakdowns' have been exactly that. I grew up with a distorted perception of the world. My thoughts about myself were very negative; I so much wanted to see myself as others saw me. I believe every time I have 'broken-down' – become psychotic – something powerful happens that, if handled correctly, can lead to re-growth. Much like cutting back a shrub, however, what has happened in reality is that my growth spurt has been stopped mid-flow.

When I was in hospital it was very frustrating. I knew if I carried on doing a certain behaviour I would discover more about me and heal. I knew I reconnected with my past at these times and relived issues that I was unable to deal with ' face to face' as they were too painful. However, in my psychotic state it was easier as there was a distance in my mind. However, this was not accepted. I remember I was reading Revelations from the Bible on the ward and I read Chapter 12. It made sense to me. It was about my life and it comforted me. When I told a nurse her reaction was that, although she could see how I made that connection, her pastor had recently been going through Revelations and said that they were very difficult to interpret. This made me doubt what I had read as

---

[2] Taken from 'Sue's Story' in Barker and Buchanan-Barker (2003) *Spirituality and Mental Health*: Whurr, London.

well as the feelings that were aroused when I read it. However today I still read that piece and it comforts me.

I agree there is a need for hospitalisation, I need a safe place to be: somewhere I would be listened to even if those around me didn't share my views; a place that I could be freer to come through psychosis without such high doses of anti-psychotic drugs. I believe psychosis is a chance for fundamental change, which is being stopped by the psychiatric system in the name of caring.

I have had 10 major episodes of psychosis and each one has been different. Each one has taught me something new about me-some things are good and obviously others are not. Over time I have also learnt to disregard what others say about my experience. They are just observers – not actual participants. Yet they are very willing to tell me what I experience.

A compassionate account of Archie's story

Variously described in his notes as schizophrenic, paranoid disorder and schizo-affective disorder, Archie might well have presented as a threatening possibility. Encountering him was quite different – modest, self-effacing, and humorous, Archie was easy to like. Given his history of repeated hospitalization under section, and the stoical manner in which he faced each day with good humour, he also was easy to respect. Archie's psychosis was slightly unusual. He didn't describe being tormented by voices and despite his long history, wasn't debilitated by 'negative symptoms'. Indeed, he was remarkably self-sufficient. His 'problem' was that he didn't belong 'here'. He knew that he existed – so he wasn't exactly suffering from a nihilistic delusion. Indeed, he knew, all to well, that he was 'here', with me and others. He simply didn't **belong** here. He was in a parallel universe, where everything and everyone was the same as the world in which he did belong. Everything was replicated down to the last detail. Only he, Archie, was misplaced – or maybe, he volunteered, he also was a 'replica'. It didn't really matter, the only thing that he could (or rather should) do, was to kill himself. That would bring this whole problem to an end, and he would, no longer, be a burden on everyone – which of course he must be, since he didn't belong here and was consuming valuable resources that, rightfully, belonged to someone else.

One day we talked about how Archie could possibly 'know' that he was in a parallel universe. With remarkable aplomb he assured me that I would 'know' if ever I found myself similarly displaced. I gave up trying the old Socratic line as he seemed wiser than any Socrates I had encountered to date and, more importantly, I felt that he knew what I was trying to do, whilst pretending I wasn't really doing anything. So began a long conversation, over several weeks, about what it was 'like' to be in a parallel universe, what kind of things he noticed, which 'told' him where he was, and how he felt about all of this. The feeling bit was the most revealing, as no one had really talked to Archie about how he felt, or so he advised me. One day I admitted, genuinely, to two things that left Archie speechless, at least for a few moments:

1. I noted how amazed I was at how 'ordinary' he was, yet at the same time he seemed quite 'extraordinary'. Before he fell silent, Archie asked me what I meant. I said, in all honesty, that I had no idea what it would be like to find myself in a parallel universe, but if I did, I feared that I might be a whole lot more disturbed by the experience than Archie appeared to be.

2. Then I added that, when I had first met Archie I thought that he was just confused about his identity. Indeed, I added, I didn't know that he wasn't, but that was another matter. Then, as we talked about the parallel universe, I realized that I couldn't possibly know that I 'wasn't' in a parallel universe. Stranger things have and do happen. (Ironically, the next day, the papers carried a story about an astronomer who said that there were probably at least several 'universes' and it was quite possible that these 'sat' next to one another, cosmically speaking. Archie didn't sound quite as 'deluded' after that broadcast).

I'm not sure if I was any help to Archie, but we got on well together. He stretched my thinking about myself: what it meant to be 'me' and what it meant to be 'here and now' – a phrase that I use all too glibly. He said that he enjoyed my company and, after my two admissions – which left him silent for a while – he reported feeling 'ten feet tall'. I could have easily said that he 'suffered from a self-concept problem', but that seemed rather obvious. Instead, I was left wondering about my own 'self-concept' after working with Archie.

Powering up practice

A core problem for people, who experience severe and debilitating mental distress, is powerlessness (Barker, 1999). Nurses need to recognise and focus upon this sense of powerlessness, providing the necessary human, interpersonal and intersubjective conditions for the development of the sense of security that the person not only seeks but needs to continue. In my clinical work I often feel like Beckett's *Unnamable,* who pondered:

> 'Where I am. I don't know. I'll never know, in the silence you don't know, you must go on, I can't go on, I'll go on.'

Such an attitude is, of course, anathema to the evidence-based lobby that appears convinced that uncertainty is an inherently bad thing. If experience has taught me anything, it is that that there are few certainties in life. What does seem fairly certain is that people like Sue and Archie have the capacity to grow through experience – even when the experience is painful. How they do this is by honing their awareness – coming to know better what they already are aware of. One of the virtues of caring is that it focuses the nurse's attention on the *person* who is the patient. Although this can impose great emotional demands on nurses, by developing their awareness of the person, there is a greater chance that the patient will develop greater self-awareness as well as awareness of the nature of the relationship with the nurse, who represents (symbolically) so many other people in the patient's life.

I found an echo of Beckett's silence in an Internet commentary on his own practice, by the American nurse and Parse scholar, Bill Cody. Speaking of his care of people in comatose states he commented:

> It seems odd in retrospect that one would have to concentrate and remind oneself continually to 'stay with' the person, hut it does require considerable dedication and effort...l found myself compelled to be fully present with the person moment-to-moment, to abide with the person in her/his unitary wholeness and focus on her/his quality of life as completely as I could. . It didn't have much to do with talking or not talking. ... It really had to do very purely and

simply with the way I was with them. Keeping the honor (sic) and respect to the fore, and really loving the person as you care for them, is the key: the rest will come.

(Cody, 1999)

Over the past 8 years my research has emphasised the need for nurses to care *with* patients (Barker and Whitehill, 1997: Barker *et al.*, 1999). We set out to explore simple questions – e.g. what did patients, and their families, and other disciplines, *need* nurses for, as opposed to doctors, social workers or other professionals? This was linked to other studies of nurses' perceptions of what they were 'needed' for, and also how they might 'empower' people who were particularly vulnerable, or distressed. The emergent substantive theory emphasised the core need for the nurse to get to know the patient, and for the patient to repay the compliment. It seems clear that we have not yet come to terms with the importance of the sense of *proximity*, which the people in our study articulated. Indeed, many of our manoeuvres in contemporary mental health care, involve distancing ourselves from patients, holding them at the end of our instruments of diagnosis and intervention, even when these are no more than form of words: the all too often malignant practice of observation being just one example (Barker and Cutcliffe, 1999).

The idea that the nurse and the patient exist across some sanity-madness divide is illusory. Perhaps more realistic is the notion of the nurse as a wounded healer (Barker *et al.*, 1996; Hall. 1996). Much of what I have done, in my efforts to 'heal' the patient, appears to have been a function of my own healing. I do something in the name of nursing that, essentially, satisfies me, but from which the person may also take something satisfying.

In the notion of nursing as craft (Barker and Whitehill, 1997) I realised that care fashions something akin to a crafted object – something with a human aesthetic quality (Skillman-Hull, 1994) that might be called an art-form, but which also depends on the exercise of some skill, or technique, that might be called a science. However, the distinctive feature of person-focused care is that the person attributes meaning to the ephemeral thing called care. Like a piece of jewelry or pottery, the crafted thing has no meaning *per se*, but is imbued with meaning through the engagement of nurse and patient.

From both a professional and social perspective, the Western world appears to be facing a crisis of confidence over its capacity to care. The insights of science have rendered us lonelier on this planet, while its progeny – technology – has made us more powerful than ever before. Science shows how insignificant we are within a universe that grinds on regardless of our efforts and suggests that our essential human experience, is no more than a genetically determined neuroscientific event (Szasz, 1996). Little wonder that people feel the need to turn to others for comfort.

Although technology might permit us to prolong life (for a privileged few), reshaping our bodies to eliminate disease, the risk we face is that the human experience that marvels at everything from the sunset and warm rain, to the Sistine chapel or the beauty of the double helix, may become redundant. Sue and Archie were *awesome* in the sense that their stories filled me with wonder. As science fiddles with the riddles of life and living, we may forget that the point of the human project is not to live without pain, far less to live for ever – but simply is to *be* and *become*. When we consider how such a philosophy might be applied to caring for those in mental distress, we might recall Epictetus' observation that 'difficult circumstances do not so much ennoble a person as reveal him'. Certainly, Sue and Archie seemed to know what Epictetus was talking about, although few of the highly-qualified professionals they encountered seemed to share their appreciation of the need for struggle in order to grow as persons.

What might be the *proper* role or function of the Consultant Nurse in mental health nursing? To me the answer seems simple: to provide the leadership and collegiate support necessary to reclaim caring as the heartland of the nursing project; to establish caring as the primary function on the nursing agenda; and to creatively develop a form of emotionally intelligent inquiry that will demonstrate that the virtue of caring also has a practical value – something that people who have known quality care, have known down the ages.

References

Allen, J. (1995) Caring in nursing: rhetoric or reality? *Professional Nurse*, 10(8), 538.

Barker P (1992) *Severe Depression: A Practitioner's Guide.* Chapman and Hall: London.

Barker, P. (1999) *The Philosophy and Practice or Psychiatric Nursing.* Churchill Livingstone: London.

Barker P (2000) Reflections on the caring as a virtue ethic within an evidence-based culture. *International Journal of Nursing Studies,* 37, 329–36.

Barker P (2001) The tidal model: developing an empowering, person-centred approach to recovery within psychiatric and mental health nursing. *Journal of Psychiatric and Mental Health Nursing,* 8(3), 233–40.

Barker P (2002) Putting acute care in its place. *Mental Health Nursing* (in press).

Barker P (2003) The Primacy of the Autologue: metaphorical reality and the attribution of self. *Nursing Philosophy* (in press).

Barker, P., Whitehill. I. (1997) The craft of care: towards collaborative caring in psychiatric nursing. In: Ti]lev. S. (ed.) *The Mental Health Nurse.* Blackwell, Oxford.

Barker, P., Reynolds, W., Ward T. (1995) The proper focus of nursing: a critique of the caring ideology. *Int J Nurs. Stud.* 32(4), 386–397.

Barker, P., Reynolds, B., Whitehill. I., Novak. V. (1996). Working with mental distress. *Nursing Times,* 92(2), 25–27.

Barker, P., Manos, E., Novak, V., Reynolds, W. (1998) The wounded healer and the myth of mental well-being: ethical issues concerning the mental health status of psychiatric nurses. In: Barker. P. Davidson. B. (eds) *Psychiatric Nursing: Ethical Strife.* Arnold: London.

Barker, P., Jackson, S., Stevenson, C. (1999) The need for psychiatric nursing: towards a multidimensional theory of caring. *Nursing Inquiry,* 6, 103–111.

Benner, P., Wrubel. J. (1989) *The Primacy of Caring.* Addison-Wesley, California.

Boon, L. (1998) Caring practices and the financial bottom line. *Canadian Nurse* 94(3), 27–32.

Bradshaw, A. (1994) *Lighting the Lamp.* Scutari Press: London.

Bradshaw, A. (1996) Lighting the lamp: the covenant as an encompassing framework for the spiritual dimension of nursing care. In: Fanner, F-S. (ed.) *Exploring the Spiritual Dimension of Care.* Quay Hooks: Salisbury, Wilts.

Buber, M. (1970) *I and Thou.* T&T Clark: Edinburgh.

Brvkczynska, G. (1997) A brief overview of the epistemology of caring. In: Brykczynska, G. (ed.) *Caring: The Compassion and Wisdom of Nursing.* Arnold: London.

Burnard, P. (1997) Why care? Ethical and spiritual issues in caring in nursing. In: Brykczynska, C. (ed.) *Caring: The Compassion and Wisdom of Nursing.* Arnold: London.

Cameron, M.E. (1996) Virtue ethics for nursing and health care. *J. Nurs. Law,* 3(4), 27–39.

Carr, J.M. (1998) Vigilance as a caring expression and Leininger's theory of cultural care diversity and universality. *Nurs. Sc. Quart.*, 11(2), 74–78.

Cody. W. (1999) True presence with people who don't speak: comments to the PARSE-L Parse Nursing Theory list: Internet 9th February 1999. E-mail: Parse-l@listserve.utoronto.ca

Cora, S. (1998) Discovering the value of nursing in high technology environments: outcomes revisited. *Holistic Nurs. Pract.*, 12(4), 31–39.

Duffield, C., Lumby, l. (1994) Caring nurses: the dilemma of balancing costs and quality. *Aus. Health Rev.*, 17(2), 72–83.

Dunphy, I.M., Winland-Brown, I.E. (1998) The circle of caring: a transformative model of advanced practice nursing. *Clinical Excellence for Nurse Practitioners*, 2(4), 241–247.

Dyson. I. (1997) An ethic of caring: conceptual and practical issues. *Nursing Inquiry*, 4(31), 196–201.

Eddins, B.B., Riley-Eddins, E.A. (1997) Watson's theory of human caring: the twentieth century and beyond. *J. Multicultural Nursing and Health*, 3(3), 30–35.

Fowler, M. (1986) Ethics without virtue. *Heart and Lung*, 15, 528–530.

Frankl, V. (1964) *Mans Search for Meaning*. Hodder & Stoughton: London.

Gaut, D.A. (1993) Caring: a vision of wholeness for nursing. *J. Holistic Nursing*, 2, 164–171.

Greenhalgh, J., Vanhanen, L., Kyngas, H. (1998) Nurse caring behaviours. *J. Adv. Nurs.*, 27(5), 927–932.

Hall, J. (1996) Challenges to caring: nurses as 'wounded healers'. *Australian Journal of Holistic Nursing*, 3(2), 12–15.

Heidegger, M. (1962) *Being and Time*. SCM: London.

Henderson, V. (1969) *The Basic Principles of Nursing Care*. International Council for Nurses: Geneva.

Holden, R.J. (1991) An analysis of caring: attributions, contributions and resolutions. *J. Adv. Nurs.*, 16(8), 893–898.

Kempe, A.R. (1994) *Forming alliances: toward a grounded theory of the nurse caring for the family caregiver of a schizophrenic member*. Unpublished PhD thesis: Wayne State University.

Lanara, V. (1981) *Heroism as Nursing*. Sisterhood Evniki: Athens.

McKee, C., Bowles, N. (1998) An evaluation of humanism as a philosophy for nursing practice in an era of rational-scientific health care. In: McMahon, P., Pearson, A. (eds), *Nursing as Therapy*, 2nd edn. Thornes: Cheltenham.

Nahas, V. (1997) Muslim patients' perception of caring. *Professional Nurse* (Singapore) 24(2), 20–23.

Owen-Mills, V. (1998) Presencing in practice: utilising the core of caring. *Aus. J Holistic Nurs*, 5(10), 4–9.

Parse, R. (1981) *Man-Living-health: a Theory of Nursing.* Wiley: New York.

Paterson, J. & Zderad, L. (1976) *Humanistic Nursing.* Wiley: New York.

Peck, M.L. (1992) The future of nursing in a technological age: computers, robots and TLC. *J. Holistic Nursing,* 10(2), 183–191.

Peplau, H.E. (1952) *Interpersonal Relations in Nursing.* Putnam: New York. (Reissued 1988, London: Macmillan).

Skillman-Hull, L.B. (1994) She walks in beauty: nurse-artists lived experience of the creative process and aesthetic human care. Unpublished PhD thesis: University of Colorado Health Sciences Center.

Sourial, S. (1997) An analysis of caring. *J. Adv. Nurs.,* 6(6), 1189–1192.

Szasz, T.S. (1996) *The Meaning of Mind: Language, Morality and Neuroscience.* Praeger: London.

Travelbee, J. (1971) *Interpersonal Aspects of Nursing,* 2nd edn. Saunders: Philadelphia.

Ward, S.L. (1998) Caring and healing in the 21st century. *American J. Maternal Child Nursing,* 23(4), 210–215.

Watson, J. (1988) *Nursing: Human Science and Human Care: A Theory of Nursing.* National League for Nursing: New York.

Yang, C., Lu, M. (1998) The effects of human caring education on nurses: a human caring knowledge, attitude and behaviour study. *Nursing Research* (China), 6(3), 206–218.

CHAPTER FIVE

When followers walk too fast

Nursing, emergent leadership and the role of the Consultant Nurse

Lyn Williams and Nick Bohannon

Introduction

The emergence of the Consultant Nurse role may present the best chance yet for nursing to play a more proactive part in providing strong clinical leadership in clinical practice and the development of clinical services as a whole. This chapter begins with an overview of where nursing began, and the journey that mental health nursing has made over the years. A key message is that the role of nursing has developed to a point where its leadership, in exploring different ways of working with clients, is central to the whole modernisation agenda for mental health services.

Walking where there are no paths – the great pioneers

A chapter that intends to look at leadership in nursing would be incomplete without at least a brief look at the contribution made by pioneering nurse leaders past and present. To discuss each of them individually would require a whole book devoted to this subject. Therefore this chapter will identify two key nurse leaders who have made a significant contribution to nursing in terms of inspiration and leadership.

Florence Nightingale (1820–1910) was a legend in her lifetime, made famous for her devoted attention to those injured in the Crimean War (1854–1856). Yet her greatest achievement was to set the standards within nursing to the level of a respectable profession for women. The Nightingale Training School for nurses at St. Thomas' Hospital was established in 1860, four years after the Crimean War. The training of 'probationer nurses' was undertaken in a period of one year and included some lectures but was mainly practical work under the supervision of the ward sister. 'Miss Nightingale' as she was referred to by the nurses, scrutinised the probationer's ward diaries and reports. Once trained, the nurses were sent off to staff hospitals in Britain and abroad or to establish nurse training schools based on the 'Nightingale Model'. In 1860 her best-known work, 'Notes on Nursing' was published and this laid down the principles of nursing: careful observation and sensitivity to the patients' needs. This work has been translated into eleven languages and is still in print.

Throughout her lifetime she campaigned tirelessly to improve health standards and her writings on hospital planning and organisation had a profound effect in England and across the world. Her vision of the future of nursing, and her reforms, have influenced the nature of modern health care and her writings continue to be a resource for health care professionals today.

Hildegarde E Peplau was another leading figure in the development and promotion of the shape and function of nursing. Famous for her work in nursing, particularly in the field of mental health, Peplau was born in Pennsylvania in 1909 and graduated in nursing in 1931. She received a Bachelor of Arts degree in Interpersonal Psychology in 1943, a Master of Arts degree in psychiatric nursing in 1947 and a Doctor of Education degree for her work in curriculum development in 1953 (Marriner Tomey & Alligood 1998). One of her most famous pieces of published work, 'Interpersonal Relations in Nursing' was scripted in 1952 and in it the notion of leadership was described as one of six different nursing roles that emerge in the phases of the nurse–patient relationship. Peplau has greatly influenced the field of psychiatric nursing and even now her work on Interpersonal Relations in Nursing offers clarity and direction to many nurses who consider the nurse–patient relationship as the bedrock of our trade.

The two pioneers described here embody the key leadership qualities to which we might aspire. They communicated their vision, they were resolute and courageous, and they enabled people to progress. These matters will be developed later in the chapter.

Standing in line – evolutionary influences on nursing

Leadership does not take place in a vacuum and at this stage some consideration of power relationships in healthcare may be useful. It is clear that imbalances in power have developed over the years and continue to exist. Service users have been disempowered and effectively cast as the passive recipients of treatment from professionals, and medical staff have been identified as the holders of the keys to information and services which has seemingly legitimised their ascent. In practice this double-edged sword has also made it harder for medical staff to truly engage with teams and clients. Specifically, three powerful cultural influences have had a significant role in supporting these imbalances in care.

Firstly, the historical tradition of the Patriarchal British culture – the medical profession has tended to be male dominated and *instrumental* in orientation, whilst nursing as a whole, was female dominated, and *nurturing* in orientation. This arrangement led to a mirroring of the oppression of females in the broader society, within the field of health care and has played its part in the creation of the inhospitable corporate cultures (Ragins *et al.* 1998) that consciously or unconsciously hamper women's access to senior positions.

Secondly, there is the issue of accessibility and influence. Entry to a medical education was tightly controlled, with relatively few places in Universities being available, and high levels of competition for these. Successful candidates would need considerable financial resources, which consolidated the creation of an elite profession.

The third factor is the reformation – with science as the new God. This notion rests on the tenet that medicine is a science, and the core belief that there was a scientific explanation behind illness that could be revealed to enable each and every illness to be effectively treated. This is a powerful and alluring proposition that potentially discounts the need to 'care'. These reductionist beliefs operate on the basis that people are little more than machines, occasionally in need of repair by skilled operators. This thinking contributes to the sense that service users should not attempt to have a voice in matters that they have not been trained in. Positivist beliefs such as these prevail today and have the 'randomised controlled trial' (RCT) as their flagship and emblematic Holy Grail.

When all is said and done, leadership inevitably involves the development of a view of what is beyond the horizon and Consultant Nurses may be well placed to inform that view. Government policy while espousing laudable aims appears to be in danger of floundering in a sea of competing priorities. In some respects it is interesting to see a government so pre-occupied with evidence from RCTs while espousing the value of the voice of the service user. The alignment process required to match up positivist data from RCTs as sought by the National Service Framework (DoH 1999) with the views of service users as experts (DoH 2001a, DoH 2001b) may simply serve to illustrate what happens when two worlds collide.

First steps – the origins of mental health nursing

The anti-psychiatry movement in the 1960s (e.g. Foucault, Laing, Szasz and Sedgwick) challenged the whole concept of psychiatry, thereby forcing it to review its origins, claims and achievements. Nolan (1993) argues that as a result of the anti psychiatry movement mental health nurses have been empowered to question why they have had only a nominal role in the historical literature of psychiatry. Nolan suggests that mental health nursing has been deprived of its founding fathers and mothers, has been left without historical role models which leaves what he calls 'a state of professional amnesia'. To some extent (since the 1950s and 60s), nursing is beginning to develop its own history with a respectable literature and tradition of theorising, researching and publishing. Reflective practice is also fuelling a great deal of writing, which again is helping to consolidate a sense of 'shared reflection' – perhaps a hallmark of a profession concerned with self-monitoring and quality enhancement.

Over recent decades, there have been major changes in the core role of the nurse, shifting through an essentially custodial function, 'containing' as it were, the anxieties of a culture. In the 1960s and 70s, mental health nurses followed the American lead in an instrumental approach, as witnessed in behavioural theory and 'token economy' regimes. The 1980s and 90s saw a burgeoning availability of nursing theory and models, and also the pursuit by nurses of training in specific psychological therapies such as Cognitive Behavioural Therapy, Transactional Analysis and Gestalt.

At intervals throughout this history, the concept of 'caring' has been of less interest to sections of the profession, seen at times as an outdated notion of not being the sort of premise upon which to base a respected profession capable of standing alongside the medics. Mainstream thinking in nursing is currently drifting towards an ever more 'technically skilled' practitioner, rather than a caring and compassionate nurse. This is creating some confusion regarding the identity and purpose of nursing, playing as it does to the aspirations of many nurses to 'develop' themselves to what they see as 'higher status' workers. The closer these nurses are able to identify with the medics, the more shored-up will be their self-esteem.

In many ways these nurses are developing their professional and technical skills at the expense of holding onto their conceptual and interpersonal skills. The person centred nature of nursing requires the ability to conceptualise life events, hopes, aspirations and traumas with a service user and to work in an honest and reflective manner. If it is likely that a process of thoughtful care may also support a process of 'humanisation' of care (Crossley 2000), then nurses may have to balance their desire for a sense of accomplishment in technical skills with the needs of service users who value the human aspects of nursing. Reflective practice does not mean retrospective practice. Thoughtful practice is reflective, but it is also proactive, creative, experimental, enthusiastic – and associated with a critical review of what is known about best practice (Wilshaw & Bohannon 2003). When seen in this way, technical skills remain a component of effective care rather than an end in themselves.

Something about nursing, especially mental health nursing attracts specific individuals into the profession as opposed to other areas of health care. It seems unlikely that an orientation towards more technical interventions figures largely in this attraction. Mental health nursing is indeed a true vocation as opposed to a career. It takes a 'special' kind of person to feel truly comfortable nursing people with mental health problems in terms of having the ability to accept the patient's experience of their illness without the security found in diagnosed diseases. Mental health nurses have traditionally resisted such 'labelling' of individuals with a mental disorder; to protect patients from the stigma associated with mental illness, and to maintain the sense of a truly personal experience that cannot be captured in a 'standardised' categorisation system. If mental health nurses cease to offer this protection and fail to instil hope into those they nurse, then the fundamental basis of the therapeutic nurse patient relationship is severely at risk.

In mental health nursing, the notions of caring, inspiring, helping and offering hope to others are strong and core principles that require nurturing through healthy nurse–patient relationships. When the nurse and the patient have established a therapeutic relationship it can be used as a vehicle to enable *hope* to be fostered with contribution by both parties. Cutcliffe (1997) claims hope is not a limitless resource because if it were no one would ever become hopeless. He recognises that if hope is considered as the final interior resource of man, hope alone cannot sustain its own existence if its energy is being used to feed and support the individual. Lynch (1965) in Cutcliffe (1997) claims that hope needs feeding and nurturing and suggests that help from external resources nurtures hope. If we accept then, that the foundation of effective mental health nursing is the nurse–patient relationship, it must follow that the nurse has a role in being able to offer hope to their patients. These basic principles have much to offer the aspiring nurse leader.

Walking hand-in-hand – nursing as part of a contemporary organisational framework

The changing role of the nurse has in many ways been prescribed by the ambitious plans of the Government. Although this seems to invest heavily in nursing, with the stated aim that there will be very different nursing roles linked to performance and accountability it seems that nurses are still too accepting of external influences that prescribe what their roles ought to be. In comparison, the medical profession has vigorously and publicly challenged many of the demands that have been imposed upon it. Although it has not always been successful, it attempts to protect the fundamental principles of its profession with passion. Nurses may need to do the same and can only achieve this with the development of a mature and reflective sense of who they are. Research, in order to build up a solid evidence base, will help – but there is a need to beware of the inbuilt bias in these processes, valuing currently as they do the positivistic over the experiential.

Margaret Thatcher's government, (1979–1990) brought to power of what is sometimes called the 'New Right'. The Thatcher government aggressively adopted monetarist economic policies and consequently viewed public services as large bureaucracies, which were wasteful, inefficient, mandatory (denying patient choice) and comfortably conventional due to uncompetitive practices (Jan-Erik Lane 1993). The 1983 report by Sir Roy Griffiths, commissioned by Margaret Thatcher (1989), called for a more effective management of the service and suggested a move within the NHS to a general management model mirroring commercial practice. This resulted in the introduction of tight management accountability, performance-related pay, performance management and target deadlines.

The Thatcher period and beyond (up until the change of Government in 1997) saw what many believe to be the slow death of the NHS. Heavily stripped by underinvestment in many hospitals, alongside the controversial changes made to the grading structure linked to nurses' pay created a sense of unrest, de-motivation and poor morale amongst nurses and other staff.

In 1997 the newly elected Labour Government proclaimed radical ideas for changes to our Health Services and made a pledge to invest in the NHS, which had been financially starved for decades. In 1997 the Department of Health produced a document titled 'The new NHS Modern Dependable', in which it stated:

> The new NHS will have quality at its heart. Without it there is unfairness. Every patient who is treated in the NHS wants to know that they can rely on receiving high quality care when they need it. Every part of the NHS, and everyone who works in it, should take responsibility for working to improve quality.
>
> (DoH, 1997)

This was the beginning of rapid changes within the NHS. The 'NHS Plan – a 10 year plan for investment and reform' laid out clear and ambitious goals, in which the government promised financial backing in return for radical improvements to the NHS. To be able to deliver on this massive agenda for modernisation it was recognised that the staff working within the NHS needed support and investment in terms of training and developing new skills to equip them to deliver the modernisation agenda. The government recognises the vital role nurses play in the delivery of care and treatment to patients. This was succinctly outlined in the publication of 'Making a difference' in July 1999, which stipulated the government's strategic intentions to strengthen the nursing, midwifery and health visiting contribution to health and health care.

It is argued that to enable this to happen there needs to be a personal and professional commitment from every nurse, midwife and health visitor. Making a Difference provides a framework for nurses, midwives and health visitors to rise to the challenges laid down within the document, to enable them to change outdated traditional practices and work in very different ways never fully considered in the history of the NHS. At the same time the government recognised that for these challenges to be overcome it needed to retain experienced, skilled nurses, midwives and health visitors at the heart of clinical practice. This document outlined the conception of the role of the Consultant Nurse. The aims of this new role being set out as essentially threefold:

1. To foster the development of clinically intelligent leadership
2. To widen the career pathway for nurses, midwives and health visitors
3. To halt the drift of experienced and skilled nurses moving out of clinical practice to further their careers via management or education.

Walking off the map – nursing leadership over the horizon

Through visiting the past and living in the present it is possible to gain a sense of the qualities that may be central to effective leadership in the future. Five key characteristics can be extrapolated from the brief account of the development of nursing in the previous sections of this chapter. These might be

1. Communicating a vision (Nightingale);
2. The importance of focusing on relationships (Peplau);
3. Instilling hope in others (Cutliffe);
4. Being motivated by a desire to humanise care (Crossley);
5. Maintaining a commitment to working towards proactive, thoughtful practice (Wilshaw & Bohannon).

These five key qualities might easily become a framework for considering leadership strategies. However we, the authors, are unwilling to sign up to the development of a simplistic mantra for aspiring leaders in nursing and the key problem with such lists is the absence of a context in which the five key characteristics should be embedded. In this case that context has the potential to be huge and all consuming. Mental health cannot be separated from other aspects of a person's life. Leadership in mental health services then might legitimately claim to have a place in every nook and cranny of each of our lives. It is easy enough to envisage a comprehensive health promotion strategy that might impact on all of our lives in many ways. Offering leadership to such a plan is a daunting task and one that will not be managed by a single leader. Rather, Consultant Nurses need to consider the context in which a problem exists and determine whether they are to be:

• The emergent leader
• The promoter of an emergent leader
• The supporter of an existing leader and plan
• The adapter of an existing leader and plan

These roles are not suggested as the only roles that might be played, or indeed the preferred roles that a Consultant Nurse might take. Rather they represent an attempt to foster a proactive consideration of the situation prior to becoming involved in order to ensure the best possible outcome for all concerned.

Being the emergent leader involves flying the flag of innovation. Consultant Nurses are well placed to undertake this duty given their highly developed clinical expertise and their functioning networks. They have the knowledge of nursing and the networks in nursing and management to ensure that they are able to innovate successfully. What individual Consultant Nurses might benefit from is some consideration of the five key characteristics identified earlier.

Promoting an emergent leader is likely to involve identifying a person who displays potential, and exploiting that potential to maximise the opportunities for development. The beauty inherent in this approach is that the person might be an emergent leader who has an idea but no authority, or has a belief but requires a more robust rationale. Suddenly there is endless potential within the workforce and the Consultant Nurse might use the four key roles to support and empower developments.

Supporting an existing leader and plan involves recognising that the world existed prior to Consultant Nurses and that each world (or service) that the Consultant Nurse enters was there before they arrived. There are of course existing leaders and plans in progress and it would be foolish to disregard the benefits afforded in the opportunity to support those innovations and their champions. The role of external supporter may be of great practical value to existing innovators.

Finally there is a role for the Consultant Nurse in **adapting an existing leader and plan.** Similarities have been drawn between managing change and herding cats and it may be that the consultant nurse will bring a bigger picture to an existing context. The gentle renegotiation of the direction and timing of a plan could easily enable it to achieve a better fit with a broader picture and lead to its subsequent success. Sometimes the obstacles that block a plan exist within its structure and an external view that is sympathetic to the overall aims of the plan can help to achieve a more balanced approach.

Central to the four roles outlined above is the notion that leadership and management should be viewed separately. Early thinking suggested that leadership was a component of management and as such, was one of a number of valuable abilities that managers might possess. In fact, while managers work with the delegated authority of the organisation to support them, leaders look elsewhere for ways of achieving their aims. It therefore becomes imperative that the five key characteristics identified earlier are present in nursing personnel who are to inspire and lead, and conversely that many of the traditional management preoccupations are not expected of them. These include budgeting, allocating resources, controlling and organising. It is our contention that there is a bias towards management rather than leadership, and that that bias represents a legacy inherited from the Thatcher years and that era's obsession with accountability and control.

If leaders are to lead, they need space and freedom to enable a high degree of creativity. Only then will they be able to motivate and enable others to take the steps from their safe and cosy current position, out into the uncertainty of new ways of being. To achieve this, leaders must communicate their vision and establish its relevance and value to others. Only by focusing on relationships and demonstrating a sound ethical basis for their actions will leaders be able to work with individuals and teams in making connections between the actions of one person and its meaning to others. As multiple smaller pictures grow into a view of a bigger world, leadership is emerging.

Evidence-based practice may be dependent on this process in order to empower practitioners to look further than their own daily habituated practice (Jarvis 1992) and incorporate the advice and experiences of others into new ways of working. Clearly being told to do it is insufficient motivation for many of us to change. Consultant Nurses are probably the most potent catalyst available to the National Health Service if they work in the manner described above. The danger, of course, is that they may be slotted into hierarchies and become artefacts of 'the system' thus clipping their wings or tying lead weights around their feet. Hopefully by attaching status to Consultant Nurses – and not management functions – they will be empowered to enable others. However it could be seen as a tempting quick fix both for managers and Consultant Nurses if a management aspect of the role were to be identified. Managers may see a benefit from having Consultant Nurses in the delegation tree created by hierarchies. Consultant Nurses may be tempted into believing that a little legitimate authority could speed things up. Both groups would be mistaken, and the only outcome would be the demise of innovation and consignment of another great opportunity to the dustbin.

The nursing role is fundamental to the delivery of the modernisation agenda and requires an organisational structure to reflect this. The emergence of National Health Service consultant posts held by nurses is an acknowledgement of the importance of nursing and the need for strong clinical leadership. It is not merely enough to support senior managers in accessing various leadership training courses. The importance of culture in mental health nursing is of paramount importance to leaders. Barker, Reynolds & Stevenson (1997) argue that nursing needs to acknowledge that the phenomena dealt with by nurses are human responses to various life problems. Those responses exist in our workforce as well. It is now time for National Health Service strategists to truly acknowledge leadership as the lifebelt for a sinking service, and for Consultant Nurses to come and stand in the light. A degree of leadership and vision are being offered at a national level by central government. However, local leaders are the people who will make a difference to the experience of receiving care. This will require creativity and if it is to be successful, leaders will need to promote thoughtful practice that aims to humanise the experience of receiving care and offer the hope of a better life ahead for all of us.

References

Barker PJ, Reynolds W, Stevenson C (1997) The human science basis of psychiatric nursing: theory and practice. *Journal of Advanced Nursing*, 25, pp. 660–667.

Wilshaw G & Bohannon N (2003) Reflective practice and whole team learning in mental health services. *Nursing Standard* (forthcoming).

Crossley ML (2000) *Narrative Psychology*. Open University Press, Buckingham.

Cutcliffe JR (1997) Towards a definition of hope. *The International Journal of Psychiatric Nursing Research*, 3, 319–332.

Department of Health (1989) *Caring for People*. London: HMSO.

Department of Health (1997) *The New NHS: Modern, Dependable*. London: HMSO.

Department of Health (1999) *Making a Difference*. London: HMSO.

Department of Health (2000) *The NHS Plan*. London: HMSO.

Jan-Erik Lane (1993) *The Public Sector – Concepts, Models and Approaches*. London: Sage.

Jarvis P (1992) Reflective practice and nursing. *Nurse Education Today*, 12, pp 174–181.

Marriner Tomey A, Raile Alligood M (1998) *Nursing Theorists and Their Work*. Missouri: Mosby.

Nolan PW (1993) A history of the training of asylum nurses. *Journal of Advanced Nursing*, 18, 1193–1201.

Peplau H (1952) *Interpersonal Relations in Nursing: A Conceptual Frame of Reference for Psychodynamic Nursing*. New York: Putman.

Wilshaw G, Bohannon N (2003) Reflective practice and team teaching in mental health care. *Nursing Standard*, 17(50), pp. 33–37.

CHAPTER SIX

Swimming with sharks

Learning about politics in health care

Mark Hardcastle

Introduction

Politics for many nurses is a dirty word. Something faceless, something beyond their control, something to do with people who have more power than them.

It's an explanation that serves the function of apportioning blame when things go wrong, when resources are difficult or when innovation is stifled. Saddled with a public image of 'woman's work' and based on ideas of nurturing, unselfish, vocational gentility its not surprising that for many nurses the murky world of politics in all its dimensions has been a place where angels fear to tread. Ironically one of nursing's icons, Florence Nightingale, was someone who was a consummate politician (Selanders, 2001). She achieved far greater things in terms of influencing health care as political lobbyist then she ever did through her clinical work as the lady of the lamp. Florence could influence, she had the ability to lead and she was granted authority. Making a Difference (DoH, 1999) hopes that Consultant Nurses will have these same attributes and lead practice developments in a modern NHS.

The role Consultant Nurses have been defined in today's NHS has been heralded as an important component of modernising the National Health Service. There has been more health and social policies introduced in recent years than in any other period of history and virtually every nurse has been touched by them. Consultant Nurses are being asked to make that difference.

This chapter will explore some of the influences that Consultant Nurses must begin to grapple with and marshal if they are to have real influence and *make the difference*. Without the power that is vested in authority it is unlikely Consultant Nurses will achieve the influences for which they strive. Gaining the authority is not a given, it's not something that occurs purely by virtue of having the title confirmed. The Consultant role is a new one, it is struggling to define itself and organisations are struggling to understand how this new species fits within their existing systems. Of course some nurses have been able to adapt – but for many learning about the politics of influence has been like swimming with sharks. This is not surprising given the large number of nurses that have been promoted to the ranks of Consultant Nurses by virtue of their clinical expertise rather than as management executives who have traditionally dictated service delivery. Let's make no bones about it – authority is about power and who has the power is about politics. John W Albarran (1995) on a rhetorically titled paper 'Should nurses be politically aware?' argued that 'being political means influencing or exerting power on others, particularly in the sphere of decision making.'

The nature of politics

Politics occur where there are differentials in power (Backer *et al.*, 1998). The less powerful you are the less control you have, and for many of the people that we work with and care about this means poorer health. Nursing espouses patient empowerment. However, the fact that we might not be very good at empowering ourselves is, to say the least, a little ironic.

Michelle Foucault, the French philosopher, was particularly interested in power and knowledge: who has it and where it came from. He said, *'maybe the target nowadays is not to discover what we are, but to refuse what we are'* (Foucault, 1982). Given nursing's probably unique potential to harness holistic biopsychosocial care, the iconography of nurses as being self-sacrificing subordinate angels must be refused if we are to develop needs-led practice, influence organisations and promote policies locally, nationally and internationally.

Society has changed since the inception of the NHS. The population has more expectations about health care, there are new technologies and there is recognition that the needs of people with mental health problems are far greater than can be met by medication alone. There is a complex jumble of psychological, medical, spiritual and social issues. A professional group that can help its clients to meet such needs ought to be a powerful influence in health care provision and not a handmaiden to a prescriber of medication. Yet as things stand, old models of care prevail without too much questioning. Old certainties will change as libertarianism gains a stronger foothold in the political landscape.

After the 1997 general election Prime Minister Tony Blair said 'the chains of mediocrity have been broken, the tired days are behind us, we are free to excel once more. We are free to build that model 21st century nation…'. Blair has no truck with 'people who say its too ambitious, sorry it can't be done. I say we are not a sorry nation. It can be done!' This was the speech of someone urging modernisation. It was as strong on consumerist expectation as it was on human rights. In the context of health care patient-centred care (not professional-centred care) is the expectation – a paradigm shift is being urged. The political markers, such as social inclusion need to be powerfully used. Nursing as a profession has a good track record of helping deliver important changes in health care, however it has perhaps not made the most of this willingness in terms of political capital (Sieloff, 1996).

Example

As a result of public concern over the community treatment of the mentally ill new legislation has been formulated as a political response to the concern. This has meant that nursing practice has incorporated the Care Programme Approach and many nurses have taken on the responsibilities of being a care co-ordinator. Nursing on the whole has embraced such changes and has shown its ability and willingness to adapt perhaps to a greater extent than other better defined and more boundaried professions. Being good at adaptation at times of change is one thing, however the power to influence such changes is another. For Borthwick *et al.* (2001) the issue is how we can combine our openness to change with influence on change is critical.

The oppression of nursing

Rather than thinking power is about coercion and domination we must realise it is necessary to use it if nursing is to be influential (Masterson &

Maslin-Prothero, 1999). Foucault (1982) recognised that competiveness for the power to secure resources leads to differences in power relations and the power of a dominant group would be able to access and secure resources over weaker groups. This might be believed to be the natural order of things. The South American revolutionary Paulo Freire, famous for his book *The Pedagogy of the Oppressed* (Freire, 1970), recognised this phenomena. Through the ability of a more powerful group to establish its beliefs and values as the 'right ones'. These would then be accepted as the norm. This could then be maintained and legitimately reinforced by the dominant group that acts in a way that devalues and oppresses groups with different values. This oppression can be seen in medical – nursing relations where to question medical opinion with a psychosocial perspective can be still viewed as anarchic. Paulo Friere discussed how important it is to 'pose the problem' and engage in processes that question the norm. To do so is to foster paradigm shift.

Swimming with sharks (Johns, 1973) means sharing the same water with dominant groups who have the ability to oppress and influence power. Swimming with sharks questions the assumed natural order of things. It means practising positive politics and becoming skilful in understanding the processes of power, the organisational anatomy, the resources, the agenda and understanding self and your reactions.

You'll only be as good as they'll let you be

Kim Manley (2000) in her work on transformational leadership, with some elegance describes a conceptual framework for Consultant Nurses that relates the role to its relationship within an organisational context. The consultant brings into the post knowledge, skill and expertise as well as their personal qualities and attributes and it is this combination that starts to operate on an organisational context.

Organisational authority should be directly attributed to the posts; it is this element of potential clout that perhaps is the single largest feature that differentiates the role from that of a clinical nurse specialist. However, if this authority is not embedded and is not capable of being operationalised in the role, it is unlikely that Consultant Nurses will impact upon the organisational delivery of services. In other words, it might be argued that Consultant Nurses will only be as influential as the organisational context allows them to be. Why should this be the case and is it possible to gain influence in such difficult waters? Traditionally, structures in health service trusts have been top-down vehicles that serve a command-control function based on hierarchy. Chief executives are supported by others at a strategic board level mostly by full-time managers. Directors of nursing may be represented at this level and whilst they may have knowledge of clinical practice they are rarely involved directly in clinical practise on a day-to-day level. Medical directors on the other hand retain a high level of clinical involvement. This might partly explain a dominance of medical staff in clinical positions on trust boards. There is therefore a danger that Trust boards are directly informed by a predominantly medical view of mental health which is taken to be the clinical perspective in the absence of other professions who are informed by a broader, more needs-led psychosocial perspective of care.

Even nomenclature is important in ensuring that Consultant Nurses have the opportunity to be powerful. The title 'Nurse Consultant' is the one that has been used by the Department of Health in the formation of these posts rather than 'Consultant Nurse' which frequently appears in academic literature, and has been adopted as the default in this book. On one level it would be petty to become embroiled in an argument about what nurses call themselves but from another stand point it is crucial as the use of language defines and is important in power relations. No other professional group currently places the term consultant after the name of their profession. Consultant Psychiatrist, Consultant Psychologist are titles that infer status and authority. Psychiatrist Consultant not only looks wrong it also implies that the post holder is someone who is predominantly consulted on issues of psychiatry only and has no other influence. Similarly the Consultant Nurse role should be far greater than being someone who is consulted on nursing issues. It is imperative that that the authority and leadership qualities of the role are inherent in the title.

Example

A group of about 30 Consultant Nurses in the South West of England, and a group of five Consultant Nurses in the Tees & NE Yorkshire NHS Trust – who meet regularly for shared initiatives, reflection, development and support -decided that they would define themselves as Consultant

Nurses. This decision was taken with autonomy and with the knowledge of bucking DoH guidance. This action whilst only mildly subversive was important in demonstrating symbolically the strength and willingness of the group to define itself and its intentions.

The disordered personalities of organisations

It is essential for nurses who want to take on a political acumen that they understand the levers, the personalities and the issues of their organisation. This can be done partly through developing emotional intelligence whereby Consultant Nurses start to think and act in ways that promote self-awareness, empathy and commitment to developing relationships based on common ground. Whilst passion and motivation may be present it'll also be necessary to control disruptive actions and manage negative feelings. Developing emotional intelligence is a development of political acumen.

In most psychological therapies a conceptualisation or a formulation of a person and their difficulties is essential in determining an intervention. A Consultant nurse wanting to develop a strategy to become authoritative in their own organisation may be served well to do the same.

The latest conceptualisations of patients who have a personality disorder stress their difficulties in maintaining relationships and have problems in being able to manage emotional distress. Characteristically, people who have some of the more severe and challenging types of personality disorder have problems with self harm, act in impulsive ways often with disregard to others, lack an ability in learning from their mistakes and an inability to reflect upon their actions, hold value beliefs and rules which are rigid, unrealistic, contradictory and unhelpful. Organisations such as National Health Service Trusts can sometimes be seen to share similar characteristics (Mulhearn, 2002) and as with some people who have a personality disorder chaos can be a defining feature. The nature of work in the Health Service is chaotic and non-linear but traditionally health services attempt to impose structure, policies and procedures that are linear in nature.

Trying to control chaos is like trying to herd cats. This might explain why despite the presence of policy and procedure manuals in wards and departments problems still arise, mistakes are made and scandals happen.

The Commission for Health Improvement and Audit (CHIA) who amongst their wide-ranging responsibilities will investigate serious incidents and will be aware of the need to examine the whole organisations and its values rather than just its policies. Whilst policies are solid tangible black and white statements about how an organisation works they do not necessary reflect custom and practice.

Similarly the apparently transparent decision making of boards and meetings starts to turn somewhat more opaque when one considers the politics of interpersonal influence that occurs in the corridors over lunch, in the pub or on the golf course. These influences are said to represent the shadow side of an organisation (Egan, 1994). Part of the Consultant Nurse formulation of their organisation must be to understand this informal shadow organisation, its politics and influences. These power relationships are fluid and socially and historically constructed. The impression is that there is *something in the water* and that it is not necessarily something tangible that drives the organisation.

Whilst it might be tempting to dismiss the shadow side as something to resist and rise above, this would be naïve because as soon as you have a group of people you have interpersonal dynamics and processes taking place. There is also something non-linear about the shadow side, unbridled by its informality it has the potential to produce creative solutions and fresh ideas that might be stifled in a more formal situation. Alternatively the resultant behaviour of the shadow side might be habitually maladaptive, ritualistic and ruled by 'the way things are done here' attitude. Part of being politically astute must be the realisation that informal relationships, rumour, brief telephone calls and e-mails contribute significantly to attitude formation and subsequent decision making. Nadler and Tushman (1988) in their influential diagnostic model of strategic organisational design describe such informal cultures as being less tangible than the formal organisational arrangements. Whilst formal arrangements such as lines of accountability and monitoring and control systems are immediately obvious they may become poor at keeping pace with altered conditions and fail to react to immediate opportunities. Informal cultures on the other hand are often more powerful than the explicit formal organisational face. Such cultures may be difficult to alter but they should never be ignored. Lack of insight into these cultures and reluctance to manipulate power have been possible reasons for our lack of influence.

Even when you are right you still feel as if you are wrong

A Consultant Nurse starting a new post inherited an operational policy for a service that was based and formulated on a model which had no evidence to support its potential effectiveness. After querying this and suggesting a service model and configuration that had some fidelity to an evidence base he received a letter from a Consultant Psychiatrist who was the Trusts Clinical Director and lead for Clinical Governance. The letter included the statement 'why should your service use evidence based practice when none of the other services have that luxury'. The Consultant Nurse felt both amazed and disappointed in equal proportions on reading the letter.

Through the introduction of new health and social policy initiatives a new health service is being visioned: one which challenges conventional orthodoxy and is charged through the National Service Framework for Mental Health to deliver services for a modern era. For many Consultant Nurses making this policy work for people with mental health problems is a prime objective.

Not unreasonably Consultant Nurses may have thought that they would be pushing at an open door when they articulated their beliefs and values around evidence based practice the development of services based on fidelity and that services would be set up with the resources, structures and support for staff to develop new ways of working.

Unfortunately the development of these services is far more complex in terms of their logistics and resourcing than many Consultant Nurses first believed and as a result Consultants may become disillusioned or frustrated. One reason may be that organisational hierarchies have difficulties in developing these new ways of working in that the staff in clinical practice are not involved sufficiently in the development of these changes.

Whilst Consultant Nurses might be articulate and possess transformational behaviours in support of modernising changes, these attributes will not be sufficient to produce the desired change without the support of the organisation. Despite wanting modernising policy to work for patients, organisational support for the introduction of modernisation can sometimes be slow due to financial, structural and cultural factors. For some Consultant Nurses this might feel like the organisation (and those that hold power within their organisation) is working against the development of modern services. Consultant Nurses must learn to understand why this is so and what might be done to minimise this resistance and increase support. For these reasons strategic skills and political 'know how' as well as knowledge, will be crucial when influencing the change agenda (Antrobus, 2001).

Some advice I would offer to assist Consultant Nurses in becoming politically shrewd includes:

- accept that in order to improve things for the people that we work with and care about as a professional you must be political
- know your turf, seize your authority and exercise your expertise. Recognise and value your expertise and its power
- be extremely knowledgeable about contemporary health and social policy and its implications.
- clarify and assess your own values and beliefs and that of the organisation.
- it's not enough to be an expert. You need to develop skills in the politics of interpersonal influence though the development of emotional intelligence.
- develop powerful contemporary networks and influences.
- listen to and get to grips with the extremely influential yet informal shadow side of an organisation.
- develop a formulation of the organisation how it works, its levers, stakeholders and it idiosyncrasies.
- pose new questions, question the way things are done 'round here', engage in processes of action and reflection.

Swimming lessons

This chapter has outlined the case for Consultant Nurses to overcome the baggage left by non-political iconography and develop an acumen of powerful influence. Acquiring this ability has been likened to swimming with sharks.

How to Swim with Sharks: a primer by Voltaire Cousteau (Johns, 1973) is a translation from French of a manuscript by the obscure author who died in Paris in 1812. It was translated by Johns, as he felt it had broader implications and uses. It was thought the essay was written for sponge divers – however it should be a reader for all neophyte Consultant Nurses. The essay recounts that nobody wants to swim with sharks but it is something that by virtue of their occupation they must do. It's a skill and must be practised in real life and it is possible to survive and become expert if some rules are followed.

- **Rule 1 – assume unidentified fish are sharks**
  Get to know the people you are working with in a wide variety of settings and situations. Learn vicariously by watching their behaviour in different circumstances. Understand what prompts them to behave as they do. What are their comfort zones and what are their likes and dislikes? Become emotionally intelligent (Goleman, 1995).

- **Rule 2 – do not bleed**
  Regulate and manage your own emotions, don't lose your head and get angry. Passion is important but petulant piques will result in injury. Exercise leadership through a transformational emancipatory approach. Avoid critical high expressed emotion in situations of conflict and frustration. Sharks will feed on weaknesses.

- **Rule 3 – counter any aggression promptly**
  Read the tell tale signs that something destructive or unhelpful is happening. Demonstrate leadership through urging reflection and a confident demeanour that is humbly authoritative. Prompt assertive action will serve to remind people of your authority. An ingratiating attitude will not be effective and can result in the loss of a limb.

- **Rule 4 – get out if someone is bleeding**
  If the organisation starts to act in a way which is self injurious or engages in cyclic behaviour where the same mistakes are replicated, get out of the water and warn every one around you. There will be failures even in an innovative environment but if life and limb are threatened

Table 1: Swimming with sharks lessons for Consultant Nurses

Rule	Essence
1. Assume unidentified fish are sharks	Know your organisation and its people
2. Do not bleed	Be emotionally intelligent, control impulsivity
3. Counter any aggression promptly	Have swagger, create a reputation as an authority
4. Get out if someone is bleeding	Don't chase lost causes
5. Use anticipatory retaliation	Be knowledgeable, be well briefed
6. Disorganize an organized attack	Divert to what is important

don't persist with something that will threaten your ability to take on future projects.

- **Rule 5 – use anticipatory retaliation**
  By being an authority, having a good knowledge of your organisation and with constant use of emotional intelligence the Consultant Nurse will be ever vigilant to power relations operating in the shadow side of the organisation. Use your strategic acumen knowledge and set the agenda.

- **Rule 6 – disorganise an organised attack**
  Demonstrate leadership by engaging in activities that are relevant in helping the organisation achieve its main objective – excellent health care. Having a vision and maintaining it, despite anxiety, using activities such as championing people and causes and strategically bringing up issues to suit your purpose. This will help to ensure that any organised attacks particularly from the shadow side can be diverted and diffused.

These rules can be summarised (Table 1 above).

Conclusion

Evaluations of the Consultant Nurse role are now starting to be published and the political dimension features. Lathlean and Masterson (2001) report that there is little evidence of power relations changing particularly with doctors. Reid and Metcalf (2001) acknowledge in their review of a

Consultant Nurse post in their Trust, that without support the role will fail. With overtones of the Hero Innovator (Georgiades and Phillimore, 1975) they accept that if the posts are set up as stand alone innovators the mistakes of the past will be compounded. Guest *et al.* (2001) in a preliminary evaluation highlight some of the problems that have been encountered including role conflicts, credibility issues and organisational and support problems as well as some success with innovation and networking amongst others. These evaluations raise many of the issues that have been highlighted in this chapter. Clearly the role is developing and the experiences and the networks developed by post holders are helping the first few tranches. For example, the Bournemouth University Consultant Nurse Learning Set led By Professor Iain Graham has developed some keys to Swimming with Sharks.

- Self-organisation
- Information management
- Understanding systems
- Developing authority
- Living with anxiety
- Relating to chaos.

Swimming with sharks doesn't mean we need to become a shark. The lesson of Orwell's *Animal Farm* should remind us of the dangers of that.

> 'Twelve voices were shouting in anger, and they were all alike. No question, now, what happened to the faces of the pigs. The creatures outside looked from pig to man, and from man to pig, and from pig to man again: but already it was impossible to say which was which.'

References

Albarran JW (1995) Should nurses be politically aware? *British Journal of Nursing*, 4(8), 461–465.

Antrobus S (2001) Growing Political Leaders. *Nursing Standard*, 15(18), 12–13.

Backer BA, Costello-Nickitas DM, Mason D, Cannon McBride A, Vance C (1998) Feminist perspectives on policy and politics. In: DJ Mason & JK Leavitt (eds) *Policy and Politics and Health Care* (3rd edn). Philadelphia: WB Saunders, 18–40.

Borthwick C, Galbally R (2001) Nursing leadership and health sector reform. *Nursing Inquiry*, 8(2), 75–81.

Department of Health (1999) *Making a Difference: Strengthening the Nursing, Midwifery and Health Visiting Contributions to Health and Healthcare.* HMSO.

Egan G (1994) *Working the Shadow Side.* San Francisco: Jossey-Bass Publishers.

Foucault M (1982) The subject of power. In: Dreyfus HL, Rainbow P (eds) *Michel Foucault: Beyond Structuralism and Hermeneutics* (2nd edn). Chicago: University of Chicago Press, 209–226.

Freire P (1970) *Pedagogy of the Oppressed.* New York: Herder and Herder.

Georgiades NJ, Phillimore L (1975) The myth of the hero-innovator and alternative strategies for organisational change. In: Keirnan C, Woodford FR (eds) *Behaviour Modification with the Severely Retarded.* Amsterdam: Associate Scientific Publishers.

Goleman D (1995) *Emotional Intelligence.* New York: Bantam Books.

Guest D, Redfern S, Wilson-Barnett J, Dewe P, Pecci R, Rosenthal P, Evans A, Young C, Montgomery J, Oakley P. (2001) A Preliminary Evaluation of the Establishment of Nurse Midwife and Health Visitor Consultants. A Report to the Department of Health. London. Kings College.

Johns RJ (1973) *Swimming with Sharks: A Reader's Perspectives.* University of Chicago Press.

Lathlean J, Masterson A (2001) Evaluation of Nurse Consultant Roles: a pilot study (Report prepared for the Wessex Medical Trust). Southampton: University of Southampton.

Masterson A, Maslin-Prothero SE (1999) *Nursing and Politics: Power through Practice.* Edinburgh: Churchill Livingston.

Manley K (2000) Organisational culture and consultant nurse outcomes, part 1 organisational culture. *Nursing in Critical Care*, 5(4), 179–186.

Mulhearn R (2002) Personal communication.

Nadler DA, Tushman ML (1988) *Strategic Organizational Design: a conceptual model for thinking about organizations.* Illinois: Scott Foreman Glenview.

Orwell G (1945) *Animal Farm.* London, Penguin.

Reid B, Metcalfe A (2001) Room at the top. *Health Service Journal*, 111(5763), 24–25.

Selanders L (2001) Florence Nightingale and the transvisioning leadership paradigm. *Nursing Leadership Forum*, 6(1), 12–16.

Sieloff CL (1996) Nursing leadership for a new century. *Seminars for Nurse Managers*, 4(4), 226–233.

CHAPTER SEVEN

Evidence-based practice and Consultant Nurses in mental health

Nick Holdsworth

Introduction

Nursing development based upon research and justified through rigorous evaluation is integral to the role of Consultant Nurse. The first public declaration of intent to create the role of Consultant Nurse was made in the document *Making a Difference* (DoH 1999). The pertinent question to address to that document is: *making a difference to what?* The pithy answer to that question must surely be *to the Quality of Care.* It is the making of a positive difference to the quality of care that all the other chapters of this text have as their cumulative end. It is also what the role of Consultant Nurse has as its final justification.

> Practice needs to be evidence based. Research evidence will be rigorously assessed and made accessible. Nurses, midwives and health visitors need better research appraisal skills to translate research findings into practice
>
> DoH, 1999, p. 44

There is a forceful reason for Consultant Nurses in mental health to be actively interested in the research, development and evaluation of nursing practice: if they are to provide effective leadership within the nursing profession, then that leadership will only be justified by consequent demonstrable enhancements to the quality of care. Only through rigorous evaluation can enhancement of quality of care be demonstrated.

There is also a special difficulty to be overcome if Consultant Nurses in mental health are to make that required interest active and effective. It is a formal difficulty (in contrast to practical difficulties, such as lack of resources) in evaluating the core functions of mental health nursing practice on a broad front (in contrast to evaluating discrete technical interventions). That difficulty is the lack of a framework within which to situate, formulate, and test nursing interventions. This difficulty arises from two sources: first, the elemental nature of much nursing activity and, secondly, the apparent lack of a comprehensive theoretical basis for mental health nursing *per se*. In consequence, quantitative research strategies leave large areas of nursing activity unarticulated and hence undervalued; they test discrete interventions but fail to capture the richer texture of the experience of delivering or receiving nursing care. The results of qualitative studies, on the other hand, are often difficult to generalise beyond the specific situation of the research itself and apply with confidence in other settings; often good at describing the breadth of mental health nursing, they are poor at framing robust justifications for approaches to nursing practice in general.

What is therefore necessary is: first, a clear recognition of the elemental nature of much nursing activity; secondly, an articulation of how the broad professional concerns of mental health nursing relate to narrower, theory-laden pharmacological and psycho-social interventions, which constitute such a small area of nursing overall; and, finally, a way of relating qualitative data to quantitative data so as to demonstrate in the strongest way possible how nursing makes a difference to mental health.

The elemental core of nursing

Nursing is an elemental activity (Holdsworth 1992). Just how elemental can clearly be seen as soon as it is realised that nursing would continue in a world in which there was no concept of cure. A world in which there was no curative endeavour would be a world much like our own, albeit less hopeful. A hospice is such a world in fact: a world in which nursing is the care of people for whom cure is not a prospect. But a world in which there was no nursing, no general care of the afflicted, would be a world in which social comity was so attenuated that no human being could long endure. So a world without curers would be tolerable; without carers, unbearable. What such thoughts suggest is that there is something distinctive and underived about nursing. It is not an occupation dependent on any prior activity, as the occupation of lawyer is dependent on the activity of legislators. Nor is nursing dependent on scientific theory, as are medicine and clinical psychology. Nursing is a response to incapacity arising out of immaturity, decrepitude, injury or illness. It is thus an anthropocentric activity grounded in fundamental human experience.

It is because nursing is such an elemental activity that the facts about it remain transparent even when the theories prove opaque, which is the true disjunction of the practice-theory gap. This transparency is displayed by the verb 'to nurse'. No other health profession possesses a cognate verb from ordinary language that denotes its function while simultaneously testifying to roots that lie deep in universal human concerns. It is also because nursing is such an elemental activity that it is so difficult to evaluate its delivery. Clarke (1999) has explored many of the implications of the elemental nature of nursing, and concluded:

> Responding to ill people with medical treatments is also to care; presumably doctors prescribe the best treatment because they think it will work but also, ultimately, because they care. To nurse individuals, however, is arguably an ethically stronger event since not motivated by the anticipated success or other specific outcomes of treatments. Nurses perceive their status as a profession to be dependant on grounds of knowledge when their worth may be more highly evaluated in respect of its moral status. It is unfortunate that we live in a society which has difficulty accepting such a proposal and of finding ways of rewarding nurses accordingly
>
> Clarke, 1999, p. 140

The logical priority of illness over disease

The starting point of nursing is an individual's self-disclosure of an incapacity or a markedly increased vulnerability to incapacity, the epitome of which is illness.

Illness is the experience of an inability readily to do what one would expect oneself easily to do and in the past ordinarily could do. The most thorough analysis of the concept of illness as 'ordinary action failure', with a specific focus upon mental illnesses, is to be found in Fulford (1989), although previous gestures toward similar accounts can be found in Peters (1960), Flew (1973) and Margolis (1975). This account can be refined into a summary definition by employing the venerable and sturdy distinction between basic actions and mediated actions (Danto 1965). A basic action is an action one does without having to do anything else, such as flexing a finger (physical act) or recalling an address (mental act). A mediated action is an action performed by orchestrating a set of basic actions so as to cause something else to come about. For example, an author moving his fingers (basic actions) across a keyboard (mediator) to write a book (mediated action): in such a case, the mediated action is described by the phrase 'writing a book'. This distinction makes basic action failure the essence of illness because basic actions are operations of self. This builds on a thought expressed by Davidson: 'we never do more than move our bodies; the rest is up to nature' (Davidson 1980, p59).

Thus, if we encounter an inability to move our own selves, then we experience illness. As a refinement of the original account by Fulford (1989), the following definition of illness can therefore be offered: 'Illness is a failure of, or impediment to, basic action(s) in the absence of hindrance from beyond the subject'.

Lack of clarity about the concept of disease and its logical relationship to that of illness riddle the literature on nursing, medicine and health care generally. It is only by reference to the ordinary-language folk-concept of illness that some biological processes become defined scientifically as diseases. The medical model is committed to the conceptual thesis that a disease is a cellular process causing organic dysfunction. What counts as a dysfunction, however, is relative to human beings' experiences and how they evaluate them. My going bald is a consequence of a biological process, but my baldness is regarded as a value-neutral state and therefore the biological process causing that state of affairs is not generally regarded as a disease. In contrast, the wastage of the body, the pain and the eventual death caused by certain forms of cellular multiplication collectively called 'cancers' are severely disvalued, and hence the cellular causal processes are regarded as diseases. In short, it makes no sense to regard a cellular process as a disease unless it has effects that human beings disvalue. Thus, the scientific concept of disease is governed by the logically prior folk concept of illness.

If the significance of this conclusion is to be properly understood, then a clear view of the respective characteristics of scientific and non-scientific explanations needs to be established. The importance to mental health nursing of establishing such a clear view arises from the fact that, just as the biological concept of disease is governed by the logically prior folk concept of illness, so the explanatory validity of scientific psychology, and the human sciences in general, is subject to tests rooted in the logically prior explanations of non-scientific folk psychology.

Scientific and non-scientific explanation

'Scientific' explanations account for phenomena by citing antecedent causes,: *'a' is the cause of 'b'* (Holdsworth 1995). The concept of cause is displayed as a logical necessity in the structure of the explanation: initial conditions are described (*e.g.* two objects, each with a mass *m* and at a distance from one another *d*); a law of nature is cited (*e.g.* the law of gravity: 'the force of attraction is equal to mass divided by the square of the distance'; usually expressed by the equation $F = m/d^2$); and then, for example, once numerical values are given for *m* and *d*, the gravitational pull between Earth and its moon follows deductively (in this case, mathematically) from the premises of the explanation.

Personalist explanations replace reference to initial conditions with talk of subjective states, such as beliefs and desires, and replace laws of nature with intentions or purposes. A person is said to have acted in a certain way because she desired that a certain state-of-affairs exist, and intended to bring about that state-of-affairs: for example, she was in Birmingham at 2.00pm and desired to be in London at 3.00pm, and purposed to bring that state-of-affairs to be by driving at 120 mph.

The point to note is that what counts as a good explanation is relative to what stands in need of explanation. Hence, not all good explanations are scientific explanations. Physics may provide a good scientific explanation of the movement of billiard balls across a baize-covered table in terms of the initial position, mass and velocity of each ball. Nothing in such an explanation, however, would convey the information required by anyone wishing to play the game of billiards. What would be missing from the scientific explanation would be the rules and object of the game.

It would be a mistake to conclude from this that the language of physics and the concerns of the billiard player are too remote to have any connection. Physics, in analysing the world in terms of atoms and fleeting subatomic particles, needs also to explain how it is that billiard balls and tables, and chalk and chairs and all the other graspable dry-goods of the universe picked out by the language of 'folk physics', appear solid and spatio-temporally continuous when the theories of scientific physics would suggest so strongly otherwise. A theory of scientific physics that failed to account for such large-scale appearances would not be regarded as adequate.

The case of the human sciences is not so very different from that of the physical sciences, except in respect of the differing origins of their respective technical vocabularies. The physical sciences of biology, chemistry and physics have evolved technical vocabularies grounded in the discoveries of objects and processes not evident to unaided observation: for example, 'atom', 'molecule', 'virus', 'cell', and 'bacterium' denote objects discovered under the microscope. The problem for the physical sciences has classically been to explain the grossly observable properties of the familiar: e.g. the stability and un-reactivity of gold, silver and copper. This is done by reference to underlying structures e.g. the eighteen electrons encasing gold, silver and copper cores of the respective atomic structures. It is this that makes them insufficiently stable to form 'electrovalent compounds' *i.e.* they do not combine readily with other elements. Hence their stability; they tarnish but do not corrode.

The case of the development of human sciences is different. Psychology in particular takes as its subject matter phenomena long familiar to human beings who, as a result, have long since evolved a subtle language in which to describe those phenomena: human experiences and behaviour. Hence, psychology has progressed: first, by re-describing the familiar and coining novel terms to denote those re-descriptions; and, secondly, by empirically testing those re-descriptions. Thus, the human being becomes re-defined: as an Operant, its behaviour 'responses' caused by the stimuli of its environment; or as an information processing unit, its sensations 'inputs' and its behaviour 'outputs'; or as a system of unconscious drives that are satisfied in increasingly remote and symbolic ways. Psychology, and the human sciences in general, re-describe familiar phenomena in the hope of discovering unfamiliar but scientifically explanatory relations holding between them.

Folk psychology

The alternative to scientific theories of psychological phenomena is folk psychology (Holdsworth 1995). 'Folk psychology' refers to that rich and extensive network of verbal accounts of subjective states and individual behaviour couched in the common language of everyday life (Hamlyn 1981; Sticht 1983; Double 1985; Miller 1992; Hodgson 1994). Its central concepts have been analysed by Swinburne (1986) and the reasons for its ineliminability, even in the context of successful mechanistic science, has been delineated by McCulloch (1995).

The elements of folk psychology are few in number, but their collective scope is great; combined, they explain a great deal.

- **Thinking** is a conscious activity using symbols, such as words and numbers; it is something one does. It is analogous to a reflex action such as breathing: an activity one is hardly free not to engage in, but over which one can have some control. The degree of purposefulness of thinking may stretch from the idle entertaining of fleeting ideas to a focused occupation with mental arithmetic.

- **Beliefs** are subjective states of varying degrees of strength that can be expressed as statements about the world. One has no direct control over one's beliefs. One cannot simply decide, for example, to believe that there are faeries at the bottom of the garden. What one can do is attend to evidence and reasoning supportive of a belief one finds attractive, and simultaneously seek to ignore contrary evidence, and thus have some indirect influence over one's beliefs. In general, beliefs are brought about by one's experiences, including the experience of thinking purposefully. One also has second-order beliefs, or beliefs about beliefs: one such would be the second-order belief that some of one's beliefs are false.

- **Desires**, like beliefs, are subjective states over which one has no direct control. A desire manifests itself as an involuntary inclination to behave in a way one believes will acquire or retain what is desired. Some desires are relatively stable, long-term wants; others are occurrent urges, such as hunger. Like beliefs, desires may be strong or weak. One can also indirectly influence one's own desires: one can reduce the urge to smoke tobacco, for example, by resisting the desire to assuage the discomfort caused by a lack of nicotine to the brain. Some desires are basic, such as the desire for food. Other desires require certain social constructions: desires for power, prestige or wealth, for example, depend for their very existence upon certain social arrangements. As with beliefs, one can have second-order desires: the second-order desire not to desire to smoke tobacco, for example.

• **Sensations** are occurrent subjective experiences and are essential to gathering information about one's environment and also about one's own orientation in space and internal physical state.

Finally, folk psychology neglects references to *causes* and to *natural laws*, as employed within scientific explanations, in favour of references to the *intentions* or the *purposes* of the human beings whose behaviour is being explained.

This behaviour may, and often does, include such behaviour as *thinking*. Thus, a person may be thinking of suicide because: she believes it is probable she will experience an event she strongly desires not to experience or is actually undergoing experiences she desires to end; and ending the possibility of any experiences, by ending her life, is more desirable than those prospective or actual experiences. This explanation does not conflict with the observation that the person concerned has a serotonergic system whose activity is below the norm, and that this relative deficiency *causes* her difficulties in recalling alternative problem-solving strategies or generating new possible behaviours she has never before considered (van Heering 2001).

Affective experiences, such as moods and transient emotions, arise from the conjunction of different thoughts, beliefs, desires and sensations. Thinking of a person, believing that person to be dead, desiring that person were alive, and having discomfiting sensations, all combine to be experienced as grief; but change the content of any one element and one changes the resulting emotion. The success of cognitive therapy, for example, rests fundamentally upon changing the content of a person's thoughts ('cognitions') and even the content of their belief-desire sets ('schemata') by which they interpret their experiences. In contrast, pharmaceutical interventions affect the content of sensations but only the processes of thinking and thus, but only indirectly, do they influence the beliefs and desires that arise from thinking about one's sensory experiences.

The personalist explanations of folk psychology thus express in ordinary language the phenomena scientific theories seek to explain. Hence, any putatively scientific explanation of a person's subjective states and behaviour must be assessed against the claims of folk psychology. Any mental health nursing paradigm must therefore rest upon a disciplined folk psychology. 'Disciplined' because it will relate to the folk psychology of everyday conversation in the same way that the crafted, economical grammatical prose of the newspaper column, novel or drama relates to the hurried, fractured, approximate chatter of the factory floor, office, street corner or shop: it is what we would say, and how we would wish to say it, if we ordinarily had the time to reflect and speak with care.

The evidence base and Bayesian inferences

The repeatability, and hence generalisation, of experimental outcomes is one of the great strengths of orthodox science. However, the practice of nursing subjugates the treatment of theoretically understood conditions, such as diseases, to the moral treatment of the person's experience of illness. This creates comparative difficulties in generalising successful nursing practices: what works in the treatment of an instance of disease D will work for all instances of D anywhere else and at any time; but what alleviates the experience of illness of person P in this place and at this time may not work for any other person or, indeed, for that same person P in different circumstances. This explains, in part, the traditional difficulty mental health nursing research has had in making a substantial impact on mental health care.

Adopting a Bayesian perspective can be enlightening as to the relative limits of quantitative and of qualitative research evidence in the area of mental health nursing (Holdsworth & Dodgson, 2003).

Bayesian probability is to be distinguished from conventional statistical probability (Berry1996). Conventional statistics conceptualises probability as the *frequency* with which a particular event may be expected in specified circumstances. Bayesian statistics conceives probability as *a measure of the strength of personal belief*, and that the strength of belief will change (increase or diminish) as more information becomes available.

Bayesian methodology assigns a probability to a hypothesis *before* any experimental procedure is undertaken. It then calculates the extent to which the experiment increases or decreases the probability of the hypothesis. While Bayesian statistical methods have been urged to inform public health policy (Lilford and Braunholtz 1996), non-numerical Bayesian analysis has been used to analyse the worth of confessional evidence in criminal cases (Matthews 1995) and more generally to analyse the grounds of rational belief (Swinburne 2001).

As an example, let it be supposed that a person with a depressive illness has recovered from an overdose of paracetomol and has now commenced treatment on an SSRI antidepressant. Conventional, frequentist statistics suggests that about half the people prescribed this type of antidepressant will show improvement in their condition (Bollini *et al.* 1999; Barbui, Hotopf & Garattini 2002); that about 1% of people who have survived an episode of deliberate self-harm will go on to complete suicide (Gunnell & Frankel 1994); and that depression carries a lifetime risk of suicide of 15% (Morgan, Buckley & Nower 1998). What all this information states about the individual is that he or she belongs to a *large class* of people about half of whom benefit from SSRI antidepressants, and that between one in a hundred and 15 in hundred will eventually complete suicide. None of this information indicates whether or not the single individual concerned will benefit from the antidepressant; that will either happen, or it will not. Nor does it indicate whether or not the individual will complete suicide; either the illness will culminate in suicide, or it will not. Thus, the evidence from randomised controlled trials and epidemiology is of limited help when applied to a specific individual.

What the nurse will be interested in, and indeed other professionals concerned with the well being of a particular person, will be the specific features and circumstances of that individual: the extent and quality of their relationships, their attitude to their suffering, their coping style and capacity for change, their expectations for the future. These and similar features are characteristically nuanced, not easy to quantify, and they are features which combine an infinite number of ways to affect clinical outcome. It is this set of qualitative facts about an individual with which the nurse will, or should, be most interested in engaging.

Thus, what starts out as *clinical evidence* drawn from the literature recedes to become *background knowledge* about a class of individuals who share a diagnosis and first-line treatment. Randomised trials, in the course of controlling for confounding factors, create a clinical nature reserve for the treatment or intervention being tested; they eliminate aspects of personality, personal circumstances, and adventitious events that have an impact on eventual outcomes.

On the other hand, what is too often regarded as imprecise clinical impression emerges in the foreground as *evidence* justifying particular interventions and nursing practices. Nurses work with individuals within the context of their idiosyncrasies, circumstances and life events.

Bayesian inference allows this reversal of the usual weight of evidence to be rigorously expressed. However, most people dislike formulae; they appear opaque and obscure. None the less, they have the merit of displaying logical relationships that hold between classes of data, and if practicing nurses are to engage in worthwhile research, development and evaluation, then an aversion to formulae is an inhibition to be overcome.

In summary, a Bayesian approach to confirmation theory calculates the probability of a hypothesis (that nursing will contribute to preventing a suicide and facilitate recovery from depression, say) as a function of *background knowledge* concerning a class of problems or type of event (suicide in depression, for example) and *evidence* specific to an individual (such as their life circumstances, the quality of their relationships, and the ease or difficulty with which they can express their distress and request or accept support).

A simple Bayesian schema would be:

$$p(H/E.B) = \frac{[p\,(E/B.H) \times p(H/B)]}{p(E/B)}$$

On this representation: 'H' is the hypothesis, 'E' is evidence and 'B' is background knowledge. Given that representation, then this algorithm displays the value for the probability of a hypothesis (say, that some person – call her Snooks – will complete suicide because of a depressive illness) as calculated by: *the value for the probability of the specific evidence*, given background knowledge and assuming the hypothesis; multiplied by *the value for the probability of the hypothesis*, given the background knowledge only; divided by *the value for the probability of the specific evidence*, given background knowledge only. This conventional Bayesian schema can be understood as a model of reasoning applicable beyond the arena of formal statistical inference.

So, p(H/E.B) asks: what is the likelihood that Snooks will complete suicide (H), given that Snooks is childless, socially isolated, and lives alone, having recently ended an eleven year relationship characterised by her being the victim of repeated physical violence and denied the opportunity to develop or maintain friendships outside the home (E); and also given that Snooks has a depressive illness, has received treatment for a paracetomol overdose taken with suicidal intent, and has recently started antidepressant medication (B)?

The answer to this is a product of three other estimates.

- First, what is the likelihood that Snooks would be childless, socially isolated, and living alone, having recently ended an eleven year relationship characterised by her being the victim of repeated physical violence and denied the opportunity to develop or maintain friendships outside the home (E); given that it were also the case that she had a depressive illness, had received treatment for a paracetomol overdose taken with suicidal intent, and recently started antidepressant medication (B) and in fact had gone on to complete suicide (H)?

- Secondly, what would be the likelihood that Snooks would complete suicide (H) given only that she had a depressive illness, received treatment for a paracetomol overdose taken with suicidal intent, and recently started antidepressant medication (B)?

- Finally, what is the likelihood that Snooks would be childless, socially isolated, and living alone, having recently ended an eleven year relationship characterised by her being the victim of repeated physical violence and denied the opportunity to develop or maintain friendships outside the home (E); given that it were also the case that she had a depressive illness, had received treatment for a paracetomol overdose taken with suicidal intent, and recently started antidepressant medication (B)?

In the example sketched, E is highly concordant both with B and with H; it therefore significantly increases the probability of H; if the data of E was *not* concordant with B (if E contained data describing a history of extensive and secure confiding relationships) it would decrease the likelihood of H. As the relationship between B and H is weak *ie* it quantifies the risk of suicide as being between only 1% and 15% the effect of E is significant on estimating the overall probability of H even though the probability cannot be quantified precisely. Furthermore, the data sketched out in E describes the scope for nursing interventions.

On this interpretation of the Bayesian schema, therefore, epidemiological and other non-personalised data – in the clinical setting, where individual patient care is at issue – constitute background knowledge, *not* evidence.

This model of inference relates the quantitative information, from the frequentist statistics to which controlled trials give rise, with the descriptive and interpretative data of qualitative studies. In doing so, it offers the possibility of displaying and rationally managing the logically different types of information which determines the character of nursing care:

1. the relative weight given to quantified clinical, epidemiological, social and other frequentist statistical data;
2. the relative weight given to non-quantified information concerning individuals and their several circumstances; and hence
3. the level of confidence invested prospectively in adopting a package of care in one context or for one person, which was originally provided with success in a different context or for a different individual.

This is therefore a technical expression of the kind of reasoning which is implicitly undertaken when considering the worth of nursing. For the broad pattern of reasoning concerning the value of nursing in any particular case is surely this: to establish the curative contribution of nursing care, subtract the speed and extent of recovery without nursing care from speed and extent of recovery with nursing care; and to establish the palliative contribution of nursing care, subtract the intensity of suffering without nursing care from the intensity of suffering with nursing care. In both cases, whatever is left over represents the nursing's contribution to the healthcare endeavour.

Frequentist statisticians characteristically object that Bayesian statistics suffers two great weaknesses: first, that it incorporates into calculations individuals preconceptions (as assumptions made as part of the background knowledge); secondly, that the outcome is merely a measure of strength of belief. The consequence of this is, in the view of its critics, that Bayesian calculations lack objective validity. The characteristic Bayesian response is that background knowledge makes explicit the assumptions buried in conventional statistical procedures, and that it is strength of belief that conventional statistical outcomes are intended to inform and which drives practical action. What is being suggested here is that the Bayesian equation may usefully be advanced as a more general model of reasoning.

Conclusion

'It is the sign of a trained mind never to expect more precision in the treatment of any subject than the nature of that subject permits' wrote Aristotle (1976 p65; Bekker no. 1094b13). It has sometimes appeared that any recognition of the irreducible approximations of accounts of mental health nursing leads to a wholesale abandonment of canonical standards of truth and objectivity (Stevenson 1996; Barker 1996). This response might be understood as a retreat into a Sophistical sulk: if these flexible rubber bands cannot reliably be measured in metres, then the metric of the inflexible 'metre' length rod is the oppressive imposition of mere convention. However, lack of available precision in a conclusion is neither equivalent to nor a licence for a lack of rigour in reasoning, including the collection, ordering, presentation and use of the empirical evidence that is appropriate to the aspect of nursing under consideration.

A clear view of the broad terrain over which the profession ranges, and the rich variety of activities undertaken in that terrain, is a necessary condition of establishing the various appropriate levels of rigour in research, development and evaluation in mental health nursing. If Consultant Nurses in mental health are to make the beneficial impact on health care that is expected, the capacity to articulate that big picture, in all its several elements, will be decisive. This will mean articulating the paradigm within which mental health nursing actually practices, and not importing into mental health nursing paradigms generated in alien arenas of activity, be they the academic pursuits of the social sciences or allied professions such as medicine or psychology. That, in turn, will mean paying special attention to the language in which people ordinarily express their experiences. It will also mean the adoption of valid and reliable models of reasoning suited to the peculiarities of nursing practice in which the idiosyncratic characteristics of the individual, controlled for and discounted in traditional large-scale research, is sometimes treated as primary evidence while the results of traditional research, usually considered to be the foundation of evidence-based practice, is relegated to the status of background knowledge. A consequence of this, for nursing, is a systematic reversal of the usual relations holding between key-concepts in health care: of illness taking priority over disease; of ordinary language taking priority over the theory-laden vocabularies of science; and of the specifics of individual experience taking priority over the generalities of clinical research.

References

Aristotle (1976) *Ethics*. (The Nicomachean Ethics translated by J Thomson, 1953; revised by H Treddennick 1976). Penguin Books: Harmondsworth.

Barbui C., Hotopf M., and Garattini S. (2002) Fluoxetine dose and outcome in antidepressant drug trials. *European Journal of Clinical Pharmacology* 58, pp. 379–386.

Barker P. (1996) Chaos and the way of Zen: psychiatric nursing and the 'uncertainty principle'. *Journal of Psychiatric and Mental Health Nursing* 3, pp. 235–244.

Berry D. (1996) *Statistics: a Bayesian Perspective*. Duxbury Press: Belmont CA.

Bollini P, Pampallona S, Tibaldi G, Kupelnick B, and Munizza C. (1999) Effectiveness of antidepressants: meta-analysis of dose-effect relationships in randomised clinical trials. *British Journal of Psychiatry* 174 pp. 297–303.

Clarke L. (1999) *Challenging Ideas in Psychiatric Nursing*. Routledge: London.

Danto A.C. (1965) Basic Actions. *American Philosophical Quarterly* 2, pp. 141–148.

Davison D. (1980) *Essays on Actions and Events*. Clarendon Press: Oxford.

Double R. (1985) The case against the case against belief. *Mind* 94, pp. 420–430.

DoH (1999) *Making a Difference: strengthening the nursing, midwifery and health visiting contribution to health and healthcare*. Department of Health: London.

Flew A. (1973) *Crime or Disease?* Macmillan: London.

Fulford K.W.M. (1989) *Moral Theory and Medical Practice*. Cambridge University Press: Cambridge.

Gunnell D & Frankel S. (1994) Prevention of suicide: aspirations and evidence. *BMJ* 308 pp. 1227–1233.

Hamlyn D.W. (1981) Cognitive systems, folk psychology, and knowledge. *Cognition*. 10, pp. 115–118.

Hodgson D. (1994) Neuroscience and folk psychology: an overview. *Journal of Consciousness Studies*. 1, pp. 205–216.

Holdsworth N. (1992) On laying the foundations for an empirico-logical model of mental health nursing. *Journal of Advanced Nursing*. 17, pp. 1095–1105.

Holdsworth N. (1995) From psychiatric science to folk psychology: an ordinary-language model of the mind for mental health nursing. *Journal of Advanced Nursing*. 21, pp. 476–486.

Holdsworth N. & Dodgson G. (2003) Could a new Mental Health Act distort clinical judgement? A Bayesian justification of naturalistic reasoning about risk. *Journal of Mental Health*. 12, pp. 451–462.

Lilford R & Braunholtz D. (1996) For debate: the statistical basis of public policy: a paradigm shift is overdue. *British Medical Journal* 313, pp. 603–607.

McCulloch G. (1995) *The Mind and its World*. Routledge: London.

Margolis J. (1975) *Negativities: The Limits of Life*. Bobbs Merrill: Columbus, Ohio.

Matthews R. (1995) The interrogator's fallacy. *The Institute of Mathematics and its Applications* 31, pp. 3–5.

Miller J. (1992) Trouble in mind. *Scientific American*. 267, p. 132.

Morgan G, Buckley C & Nowers M. (1998) Face to face with the suicidal. *Advances in Psychiatric Treatment*. 4, pp. 188–196.

Peters R.S. (1960) *The Concept of Motivation*. Routledge & Kegan Paul: London.

Stevenson C. (1996) The Tao, social constructionism and psychiatric nursing practice and research. *Journal of Psychiatric and Mental Health Nursing* 3, pp. 217–224.

Stitcht S.P. (1983) *From Folk Psychology to Cognitive Science: The Case Against Belief*. MIT Press: Cambridge, Massachusetts.

Swinburne R. (1986) *The Evolution of the Soul*. Clarendon Press: Oxford.

Swinburne R. (2001) *Epistemic Justification*. Oxford University Press: Oxford.

Van Heering K. (ed.) (2001) *Understanding Suicidal Behaviour*. John Wiley & Sons: Chichester.

CHAPTER EIGHT

Qualitative research method
A guide to the Consultant Nurse researcher

Gary Wilshaw

Introduction

The purpose of this chapter is to explore the thinking behind qualitative methodology in nursing research, a paradigm that I believe to be of crucial importance to mental health nursing and the role of the Consultant Nurse. In particular I shall look at the processes and methods of grounded theory, an important and relevant method of understanding social/interpersonal phenomena such as those found in emotional suffering.

A crucial part of the intention of this chapter is to articulate clearly the beliefs and assumptions that underlie the qualitative paradigm, in order that the reader can make an informed judgement concerning both published work, and the design of any enquiry that they may be considering. As a background or starting point, the immediately following sections will review key influences within social/interpersonal enquiry. I do not intend to offer a clear cut, black and white definition of the fundamental philosophies because it does not seem to me that any approach is constructed in that manner. More likely, there may be as many approaches to qualitative research as there are qualitative researchers, such is the value ascribed in contemporary work of this type to the role of the *individual* researcher in giving authorship of meaning in social or interpersonal phenomena.

However, any formal enquiry into a phenomenon must necessarily be guided by a set of beliefs, be they implicit or explicit (Guba, 1990). Ideally, these beliefs will guide the reader or researcher, by offering a view on the nature of knowledge or reality (ontology), the relationship between the researcher and the knowledge (epistemology) and how to go about unearthing or giving authorship to knowledge (methodology).

Qualitative and quantitative approaches in mental health nursing: an outline

Positivistic, quantitative approaches

In the field of mental health nursing research, there is a tradition of the influence of the medical profession (Pearson, 1992), which itself was heavily influenced by the research methods of natural science. A consequence of this has been the permeation of positivistic ontology, epistemology and methodology into mental health nursing research, reflecting the biomedical basis of Western medicine and a basic belief in a relatively simple cause-and-effect view of relationships between 'variables'. Ontologically, this paradigm suggests an objectifiable 'truth' or indicator of a universal law that organises the world and our experience of it (Guba & Lincoln, 1998). Flowing from this, there is a tradition of attempting to establish somewhat linear relationships between phenomena – promoting a dominant epistemology of 'knowing that' rather than 'knowing how' (Cutcliffe, 1998). McKenna (1997) has argued that this has been problematic for nursing and that it is not enough for a profession that is essentially practice based and action oriented. Indeed it may be that the historical and still influential positivistic paradigm has supported what is often referred to as the 'theory-practice gap' (Cutcliffe, 1998), with a knowledge of 'know-how' lagging behind the knowledge of 'knowing that'. Research information emanating from within a positivist paradigm is commonly numerical, or concerned with the establishment of quantifiable 'facts'.

Methodologically, the 'randomised controlled trial' (RCT) is by far the most favoured research method of the quantitative paradigm in mental health nursing. Many prominent contemporary mental health nursing researchers (e.g. Moody, 1990; Gournay & Ritter, 1997; Brooker *et al.*, 1994) attempt to persuade readers that the RCT is the only true way of establishing the 'truth' about the effect or value of an intervention in nursing. This illustrates further key tenets of the belief system:

- that there is a *controllable/pliable* set of variables operating within (or upon) the phenomenon
- that these variables can be objectively observed
- that they can be *measured* as they vary

- that repeat measures will subsequently see the variables behave in the same way (reliability)

The philosophical position that encourages the search for *the* truth, is sometimes referred to as the *realist* position. Within the paradigm, there is an ontology that there exists a singular reality out there, 'driven by natural laws' (Guba, 1990, p. 19). In mental health nursing research, workers with this orientation are likely to be addressing questions around the notion of 'what works?' and would typically be attempting to measure the response of the client to a given treatment or intervention on the part of the nurse (e.g. Brooker et al, 1994). This approach is very much modelled on the way pharmaceutical companies might set out to measure the efficacy of a new drug, using the principles of the double-blind RCT.

While this research paradigm brings with it a certain credibility from a long and dominant history, it can also be criticised for being an unsuitable a way of learning about the lived experience of people, or indeed the social/interpersonal world of mental health nursing and of the therapeutic relationship. Barker (1997b) argues that as a result of pressure to work with a positivist paradigm, the essentially 'holistic' nurse is overcome with anxieties about what does and doesn't 'work':

> … many nurses have committed themselves to the idea of a marriage of holism and psychiatric technology…
>
> (Barker, 1997b, p. 19)

As a result of this kind of pressure, it may be that nurses are being encouraged to 'atomise' (Dawson, 1997) both the client's and their own experience of either emotional distress or the process of helping. At the same time (and hence the anxiety) nurses place great store on the principles of holistic care and the recognition of the uniqueness of the client as an individual.

Similarly, Benner (1984) argues that it is the knowledge embedded in mental health nursing that needs to be illuminated in order that it may produce theory that is appropriate to supporting creative and helpful nursing practice. She argues that this knowledge is not accessible using quantitative methods or approaches. This may be particularly the case when the focus of enquiry is concerned with, for instance, the experience of distress or the perceived value of the therapeutic relationship. A difficulty may be, then, that a research paradigm that depends upon measurement and quantification, may become interested only in that which is conveniently measured.

The qualitative paradigm

To some extent, the emergence of a qualitative paradigm may be seen as a reaction to the sort of positivistic dominance in mental health nursing described above. The key advantage of a qualitative approach for research into a given phenomenon is the depth and complexity of exploration that it affords. The generation of rich or 'thick' data (Geertz, 1973) allows for the discovery of *meaning* that cannot always be anticipated or hypothesised about. There is less assumption of an *objective* reality and instead the researcher is concerned with the discovery of *meaning*, often the subjective meaning, ascribed by the research informants. Guba suggested that instead of a unifying *objective* reality, there is a sense in which reality is individualistic or relative:

> ... realities exist in the form of multiple mental constructions, socially and experientially based, local and specific, dependent for their form and content on the persons who hold them.
>
> Guba (1990, p. 17)

The discovery of knowledge then, is here more concerned with situation specific authorship of ascribed meaning to the phenomenon, rather than a claim to a *universal* truth.

The increasing interest in the use of naturalistic enquiry has led to the development of several meta-paradigms that all fall under the umbrella term of qualitative research. These include phenomenology, critical theory, ethnography and grounded theory. I shall describe each of these meta-paradigms later in this chapter. For the researcher, after clarification and identification with the key tenets of the qualitative paradigm, it is important to orientate oneself using these meta-paradigms, using their epistemological features as reference points.

Whereas quantitative methodology is sometimes thought of as a *deductive* approach to enquiry, qualitative research is often thought of as *inductive* or interpretative. This is false dichotomy however, as it may be perfectly reasonable to *induce* conclusions from any form of data –

including numerical. A *deductive* process is usually concerned with the derivation of theory from other, pre-existing theory – often by testing an idea or approach in a novel situation.

Inductive processes require an interpretation of data that is free from assumptions of what will be found (*a priori* theory) in order to construct theory. In doing this, allowance is made for the distortion or bias of either the informant, the researcher or both. The data certainly informs the construction of theory, but this can only be done through the *reading* of the data, along with '… the assumptions of the researcher about the nature of life, the literature we carry in our heads, and the discussion we have with colleagues' (Strauss & Corbin, 1998, p.137).

Reflections of the development of this alternative, naturalistic paradigm are also found in mental health nursing, counselling and psychotherapy *practice*. Just as the medical profession has influenced thinking about research and methodology, so has it influenced thinking about the nature of emotional, socio-emotional distress or 'mental illness'. The influence here has been to promote a diagnosis-then-treatment, and somewhat reductionist approach. An alternative paradigm has encouraged a view that emotional distress may also be (at least in part) individualistic and have meaning that relates to the highly unique life of the individual. This belief will then of course support an approach to the conduct of therapeutic relationship that is more concerned with focusing on the experience of that individual, moving into their worldview and providing help when having gained the concomitant understanding (Burnard & Hannigan, 2000).

Mixed paradigm models

Arguably, it is unhelpful to split quantitative and qualitative paradigms as if they are mutually exclusive. Perhaps because of a reaction to the domination of positivism in mental health nursing research, some researchers in mental health nursing appear to place themselves firmly in the qualitative camp and eschew quantifying methods (e.g. Barker, 1997a). The adoption of such a position is understandable as a means to establish an approach, against a backdrop of resistance from prevailing ideologies.

The earliest shifts from positivism however, allowed post-positivistic researchers to legitimately mix the principles of the quantitative, experimental model with qualitative natural inquiry perspectives (Hill-Bailey, 1997). These researchers seem to approach their work, with the belief that there is a realist knowledge 'out there' in the social world that can be best understood with a blend of the two approaches.

I have already mentioned the importance of researchers orientating themselves to the values of the method chosen. This may mean that it is problematic for some researchers to adopt a 'mixed method' approach, without compromising values or belief systems. Presumably the 'real world' of research is characterised by an untidy or eclectic blend of ideas, which roughly approximates the untidy nature of the human experience.

The methods of the qualitative paradigm

It is important to recognise that the intention of qualitative research is, as stated, to give *authorship* to meaning and to contribute towards an understanding of the highly complex, multi-faceted, ever changing nature of human behaviour and human experience. Because of this, an approach to qualitative research methodology is needed that will allow this complex world to 'express itself'.

Somewhat paradoxically perhaps, Hill-Bailey (1997) suggests that the move in mental health nursing to an interest in qualitative methods, represents what could be seen as a simplification of research thinking. What she means is that the fundamental stance of the qualitative researcher is to look, to try to understand, and to be essentially open about this process. She argues that this is, in some ways, uncomplicated behaviour. However, while there may be uncomplicated surface behaviour in the researcher, the processes at work in analysis are, in my opinion, perhaps *more* sophisticated than the quantitative equivalents of numerical manipulation.

In qualitative research, the relationship between the researcher, the informant and the data is often quite significantly different than in quantitative work. Strauss and Corbin (1998) report that many qualitative researchers report feeling 'changed, beneficially' (p. 4) after undertaking qualitative research, signalling to me an important inter-relational *developmental* pathway that seems inherent in the paradigm. Elsewhere in this text, both Phil Barker and Mick Norman both, in their own ways, refer to processes where the receptive nurse may grow and develop as a result of their openness to the experience of the person who is suffering. Rather than an instrumental and aloof approach to the study of the 'subject', the qualitative researcher may *work with* 'participants' or 'informants'. These semantics suggest a much more mutual process of exploration of meaning that may well have an impact of some sort on all participants – including the researcher. The *complex* behaviour of the researcher then, is more likely to be seen in the skills applied to the very process of working with informants as collaborators of some sort, and also in the *thinking* about the data gathered. However, this is *not* to suggest or claim that qualitative researchers are somehow always 'nicer' than their quantitative colleagues. Even the infamous Rosenhan (1973) study – 'being sane in insane places', whilst essential qualitative, was of course deeply deceptive. More recently, Clarke (1996) went to great lengths to conceal the fact that he was researching the culture on a mental health secure unit, including masquerading as a nursing assistant, and feigning newspaper reading whilst actually listening to conversations between staff on the unit.

Approaches to data generation need to be creative and flexible and give maximum opportunity for the phenomenon to reveal itself. This means that the researcher needs to be reasonably *comfortable* with ambiguity, be willing to *explore* that ambiguity, and be able to resist the urge to quickly achieve closure or analytically neat results (Strauss & Corbin, 1998, pp. 5–6). Instead, qualitative research methodology is characterised by a relatively naturalistic gathering of data, followed by analysis, followed by further data generation and so on. As this process proceeds, supporting or conflicting evidence is added to an increasingly rich tapestry of meaning and depth.

Analysis of qualitative data

An assumption in the analysis of qualitative data, is that there is order and meaning there that can emerge, given the opportunity (Marshall, 1981) and appropriate conditions. As I have remarked earlier, the process of qualitative research is concerned with giving an authorship to such order or meaning, in a way that communicates both its essence and its complexity.

Analysis is a personal process, and there is no claim that the researcher's personality is not interwoven with the findings and the methods used to work with informants. These features are declared however, and therefore *available* for the reader to take account of in their own thinking about the research.

The analysis of data in qualitative research is concerned with the search for patterns, qualities and meanings, via processes of observation, immersion, de-construction, re-construction, synthesis, elaboration, reflection and others (Sanders & Liptrot, 1994). Coffey & Atkinson (1996, p. 6) encourage qualitative researchers to 'play and experiment' with data, supporting ideas put forward by Tesch (1990, cited in Coffey & Atkinson) concerning the multiplicity of ways of approaching qualitative data.

Handling data may be a process-oriented activity, perhaps concerned with indexing, counting and the de-construction, say, of interview transcripts. Alternatively, qualitative data analysis may focus on imaginative and creative interpretation as a means to encourage a range of perspectives in looking for meaning. For example, in one piece of my own work, I worked with survivors of childhood sexual abuse to explore the lasting effects of this upon them as adults. One approach I used to do this was to invite these individuals to paint pictures, select and share favourite music, to write poetry and then to look at this creative process (and product) with others, in a small group. By looking at the work created, associating with it and 'playing' with the ideas (for instance in psychodrama or role-play) an opportunity was created to look at meaning and the lasting impact of early traumatic experience.

In the example given, data generation and analysis occurred in the group setting and was a shared activity. My own individual analysis was conducted privately but then taken back to the group to be shared and modified in the light of the opinion of these partners in the exploratory process.

Meta-paradigms within qualitative research

There are, of course, various approaches *within* qualitative research that shape the way a study is conducted and conceived. These approaches include grounded theory, phenomenology, ethnography, critical theory and emancipatory research. The list is quite long and sometimes confusing, in part because of the sometimes subtle use of semantics. Put simply, each approach, brand or individual adaptation of qualitative research may be characterised by the degree to which it embraces a positivist, interpretative or critical theory stance. I will now take a brief look at each of these paradigms with the aim of demonstrating that each may influence any form of qualitative research, and that no approach is a product of purist thinking.

Positivism

Commonly thought of as a quantitative research philosophy, it is also true to say that qualitative research may often have positivistic influences. On some occasions, I have had the impression that the basic standpoint even of Strauss and Corbin (1994), suggests a certain realist stance, as witnessed in expressions like '...studying social reality' (1994, p. 4) although I guess that they may reject a positivistic label.

Interpretivism

This is embraced and perhaps best illustrated within phenomenological research, which has its roots in social psychology. Workers who hold this philosophy do not see it as possible to perceive, collect or analyse data in an objective or in any sense 'removed' manner. Phenomenology can be thought of as attempting to understand the nature of being, or lived experience through the window of language (Hill-Bailey, 1997). The task of this researcher is to attune to the subjective reality of the informant, and to attempt to describe the very essence of 'being' as seen from the informant's viewpoint. Usually, phenomenology presents interpretations (rather than theories) of experiences and attempts to allow for the researcher bias or perceptual filters by acknowledging and describing these, rather than trying to 'control them out' as a positivist researcher would.

Concern about the accuracy of interpretations made sometimes leads to an emphasis on discussion of the meanings given to certain words or phrases used by the informant, in an attempt to anchor interpretation in an almost concrete observation from the field of study.

Critical theory

This is a political philosophy that has an agenda of emancipation of an oppressed cause or group. A good example of research traditions that have powerful influences of critical theory would be feminist research and the feminist influence on research philosophy in general.

Early feminist research held that the 'objective', positivistic stance is essentially masculine and instrumental and that it reflects a dominance of the male upon the progress of scientific enquiry. Typically, this criticised stance is such that the 'self' of the researcher is separate and aloof to the 'subject', reflecting an unequal power base similar to that of male domination over aspects and exploitation of nature. Attempts to foster objectivity are seen as further alienating the 'subject', who becomes an object to be 'manipulated', 'controlled' or 'measured'. Feminism has influenced nursing research (Williams, 1990) and the increasing desire to involve patients/clients as colleagues in the research process.

Critical theory can be incorporated into any qualitative method to varying degrees. Although it may be fair to point out that the desire to empower and emancipate the participant will rarely go as far as it might in a theoretical sense. This is because the researcher will usually retain an 'advantage' in terms of biography, ability to publish papers and so on, which helps support quite different relational position and power balance between the 'researcher' and the 'researched'. Clearly though, the influence of critical theory has powerfully shaped methods that respect and value the informant as *near* equal. The stance, at least, allows for involvement of the informant in study design, data generation and analysis as an active partner.

Grounded theory

As a form of naturalistic enquiry, grounded theory was first articulated by Glaser & Strauss (1967) and is represented in contemporary mental health nursing related studies in modified forms (e.g. Cutcliffe, 1997; Jackson & Stevenson, 1998; Coyle, 1999). This approach shares some of its qualities with other qualitative approaches, such as the principles of interpretivism, methods of data collection, and an intention to give authorship to subjective and unique realities of informants. The latter point perhaps reflects a thread of phenomenology to a greater or lesser extent.

What is different about grounded theory however, is the emphasis placed upon a systematic analysis leading to *theory development* (Strauss & Corbin, 1994, p. 274). This is especially useful when little is known about the phenomenon being researched, where key meanings and issues are allowed to *emerge* from the data and point to theory development (Simmons, 1995). Strauss (1987) asserted that grounded theory is not of itself, a specific method or technique of research. Instead, it is a style of doing qualitative research that has particular approaches and techniques within it. Included among these techniques are open and axial coding, theoretical sampling and a process of 'constant comparisons' (Strauss, 1987, p. 5). This view is challenged by McLeod (2001) who suggests that the earlier Glaser & Stauss works on grounded theory looked *distinctly* procedural, methodological and had little to say about the relationship, exploratory or otherwise, between the researcher and informant. McLeod's (2001, p.71) view is that some strands of grounded theory thinking can be accused of a 'downplay' of collaborative working, such as is highly valued by feminist research for instance.

In essence, the process of analysing data using the principles of grounded theory involves, among other things:

- facilitation of the emergence of theory
- coding or inductive interpretation of data
- exploration of the features and dimensions of that coding
- grouping or 'categorising' of codes that form a cluster of meaning
- filtration of data by a researcher with a 'free floating' attention to detail and possible meanings
- movement from concrete to the abstract and back again, testing and comparing how well abstractions help illuminate meaning
- experimenting with connecting new meanings to existing research findings, to explore links, conflicts and supportive ideas
- memo writing, journal writing and diagramming by the researcher, as a means of continuous reflection and checking/recording of thought and feeling development
- openness to interpretative possibilities that are unexpected
- self-awareness of bias and 'interests' in the researcher
- use of the self of the researcher as a sensitive instrument to *notice* and accept internal and external observations.

Grounded theory depends upon the use of empirical *indicators* of the presence of concepts in any given data set (Strauss, 1987). Such indicators are pieces of data that point to the existence of a concept or category of meaning, at first tentatively and as the process goes on, with more (or less) certainty. As this occurs, weight is added to (or subtracted from) to the validity of the concept. If many indicators emerging from the data stand the process of mutual comparison and continue to point to the presence of the concept, then the beginnings of theory may take root. This process of mutual comparison, is concerned with looking at similarities and differences embedded in the data that may suggest a level of comparability that may justify a *grouping* of the indicators to support the theorising of the presence of the given higher-order concept.

Following from this, the newly emergent concept is checked back against the *specifics* (returning from the abstract to the concrete) to see how the two 'sit' together. In this process:

> ... concepts ... have earned their way into the theory by systematic generation from data ... conceptual specification is the focus of grounded theory ... because the operational meaning of the concept derives from the use of its earned distinctions in the grounded theory.
>
> (Strauss, 1987, p. 26)

Here, Strauss is emphasising that the rigour inherent in grounded theory, is due in large part to this process of theory development that is firmly and demonstrably embedded in a data-base. This process was *especially* important to Strauss and colleagues, who developed grounded theory at a time of much criticism of qualitative methods because of a sometimes less than clear pathway or paper-trail, that showed where interpretations had come from. However, the qualitative researcher needs to be aware of the risk of adopting a somewhat defensive stance in this respect, and adopting so-called 'objectified' strategies in an unhelpful attempt to gain a form of credibility sought traditionally by positivists. Similarly, Johnson (1999, p. 68) cautions against what he calls 'the qualitative drift to positivism' and the potential loss of creativity, a vital ingredient in qualitative research.

This point raises a tension apparent within contemporary deployment of the principles of grounded theory. To remain philosophically true to itself, this qualitative method seeks not to be 'representative' or 'standardised' in any form. Instead, an interpretation (albeit transparent) of meaning should be offered, which may draw upon rich and highly subjective process of thought, feeling and interaction within the researcher and the relationships with his or her informants. However, in their later work, Strauss & Corbin recommend that:

> Given the same theoretical perspective of the original researcher and following the same general rules for data gathering and analysis, plus a similar set of conditions, another investigator should be able to come up with the same theoretical explanation about the given phenomenon.
>
> (Strauss & Corbin, 1998, p. 251)

Johnson (1999, p. 69), goes so far as to suggest that this sort of thinking represents 'nothing less than a form of inter-rater reliability', which would seem to be at odds with the interpretative roots of the tradition. Given that this message has come from the highly influential founding figures of grounded theory, one may reasonably assume that the influence risks widespread contamination of what might be a truly alternative paradigm to positivism. Morse (1997) advocates the deployment of methods of evaluation of research that are appropriate to the sort of theory it *intends* to generate. Morse would agree with Johnson (1999) that qualitative researchers may be guilty of being too modest about their findings, and may compound this by resorting to the use of evaluative paradigms from the quantitative world.

It is of interest to note that there appears to be a significant difference in the way the two principal founding figures of grounded theory approach its use from a deep philosophical level. Denzin & Lincoln (1994) suggest that grounded theory is compatible with a *rational* and modern approach to science – suggesting perhaps, this is why it has proved to be so popular, and also perhaps that the reason for its popularity is its palatability to those of a more positivist/rationalist/realist persuasion. This procedural and sometimes over-systematised 'feel' of grounded theory, remained a characteristic of the work of Strauss until his death in 1996, and through his collaboration with Juliet Corbin (e.g. Strauss & Corbin, 1998). Strauss (1987) would contest this though, as he justified his approach as providing 'rules of thumb, not rules' (p. 7).

Personally, I would say that my reading of Strauss has had the sort of influence implied in the latter quotation, but this may be accounted for by my personal biography and some confidence in collaborative working practices. A further argument, as McLeod (2001) says, is that if a professional studies his or her own profession, (nurses studying nursing) the deep familiarity may facilitate the sort of *absorption of principles* I refer to.

In contrast to the influence of Strauss, Glaser (e.g. 1978, 1992,) has emerged as representing a model of grounded theory that might be thought of as remaining more philosophically true to the qualitative tradition – even contributing to its *development* and maturation. Glaser (1978) wrote of emergent, as opposed to forced theory development in grounded theory. This perhaps captures the key difference between Strauss and Glaser, that of Strauss's sometimes *procedural* response, to achieve acceptance in contemporary science, versus the more *intuitive* Glaser, who might be more willing to remain more phenomenologically oriented.

This pull in two directions witnessed in the styles of Strauss & Corbin as individual writers and key figures in grounded theory, is also witnessed within the influential work of Morse (e.g. Morse & Field, 1995; Morse, 1997) in nursing research. In 1995, Morse and Field advocated that qualitative findings should, if they are to be of value, be able to stand up to the rigor of 'quantitative testing' (p. 10). This assertion by a much respected writer might have been seen as something of a serious compromise of the phenomenological/'Glaserian' influence in grounded theory foundations. Sure enough, this is fully acknowledged by Morse (1997), when she recommends that readers who own her 1995 co-authored text '…tear out the page…' that gives this advice! Morse's (1997) view is that there is danger in becoming too focused on *method* in qualitative research, and that we risk 'missing' how useful, informative and helpful findings often are.

And so it is with this debate in mind, that I shall now outline some of the procedural and analytical structures that are used and adapted in grounded theory, that help achieve the data-embedded theory development described. At all times, *this* researcher/practitioner remains aware of these procedures, in a way that allows for their adaptation and infusion into an essential collaborative and exploratory venture with informants, which demands reflexivity and a capacity to respond to what is happening in an immediate and dynamic sense.

Coding

Coding basically refers to a process of assigning 'tags' or labels to pieces of data (interview transcripts, field-notes, artwork or whatever). These 'pieces' can be single words, sentences or larger sections. The point of this exercise is that the code helps attach some sort of *meaning* to the piece of data, either at a fairly concrete or 'indexing' level, or at a more abstract level. It is in some ways a process of data reduction (Miles & Huberman, 1994) that begins the larger process of re-construction into meaning and theory.

In the former of these two approaches, the researcher may feel it is useful to simply note and label the occurrence of certain vocabulary. Coding in this manner remains at the concrete level, but can contribute to the construction of meaning by enabling an almost quantitative feature of data manipulation into the equation. Coding that in some way attaches a more abstract meaning to a piece of data, can be seen as an initial step in conceptualising or analysing the data, although some writers are keen to point out that coding is not a *substitute* for analysis (Coffey & Atkinson, 1996). It seems to me that there is a degree of analysis beginning, because the researcher is actively *doing something* with the data that in a way *changes* it by decontextualising it. Once this decontextualising is done, and a (relatively) abstract code is attached, the data segment is as it were 'opened up' to the possibilities of re-connecting it to new interpretations, meanings or contexts.

The reason Coffey & Atkinson (1996) are cautious about the function of coding, is because its prime role is to help marshal data segments into clusters or categories, containing data that does (or does not) have a common thread. This could be conceived of as primarily a practical task, rather than an analytic one. However, my experience is that the sort of *thinking* that can accompany the coding procedure, is often a creative one that can feel much *more* than the simple assigning of tags or labels. The segmenting and grouping of data in the coding process may be done by hand, using cards, coloured codes and so on, or may be assisted by one of several computer software programmes now available. Software is still concerned with organising and retrieving data however, and in no way contributes to the process of analysis, other than by facilitating ready retrieval, searches, storage of data and so on. Well known software packages include Atlas.ti; NU*DIST; and Ethnograph.

It is not really possible to separate coding from analysis for other reasons. One of these is that analysis does not *wait* until coding is complete. Analysis may occur simultaneously, as the researcher begins to note and become sensitised to emergent meanings. This sensitisation may then influence subsequent coding. In addition to seeing coding as data reduction or simplification, it can also be seen as data complication (Coffey & Atkinson, 1996). The process of coding can add richness of meaning and open up interpretive possibilities, use of metaphors or conceptual contradictions.

Coding: micro or macro treatment of data

Coding of data segments may be applied as a result of *asking questions* of the data at a *micro* or more *macro* level. My experience is that I have regularly switched from one to the other, looking at how the *answers* to the questions compared.

Microanalysis involves a line-by-line scrutiny of the data, looking at the words and sentences, choices of vocabulary, common or less-common meanings and so on. Many techniques can assist this extremely laborious process, including what Strauss & Corbin (1998) refer to as the 'flip-flop' technique (p. 94). Here, words are played with, turned into opposites or extremes, in order to help illuminate the properties and dimensions of the word or phrase. If we explore the meanings of 'weak' or 'super-human-strong', opposites and extremes of meanings may emerge. This may then facilitate the uncovering of the *properties and dimensions* of the original 'strong'. A process close to this is referred to by Strauss (1987) as *axial* coding, referring to an exploration of the *axis* or dimensional properties of a specific category meaning.

Coding in a *macro* sense, refers to the attachment of a descriptive or analytic tag to a larger segment of data – say a paragraph or page for instance. In this form of coding, the attached code may well be the researcher's attempt to make an early comment in response to the question 'what is going on here?'. The code may capture something of the *essence* of possible meaning in the segment, and may be more likely to be at an abstract level.

Open coding

In many ways, the process of coding represents the interface between the data and the researcher (Strauss, 1987). The code clearly *comes from* the researcher. It is a concept that *belongs* to the researcher, in that he or she has, albeit tentatively, attached it to the data segment as a result of it triggering a response in his or herself. Until subsequent support or conflicting meaning is unearthed, this remains a singularly and deeply subjective act. It is for this reason that the researcher needs to bring a good degree of self-awareness to the process, or what Coffey & Atkinson (1998, p.59) refer to as 'self-conscious … discipline'. Personally, I feel that 'self-conscious' is a less useful concept in this context than 'self-aware'. The former implies to me a discomfort and unease, which I believe may in fact hinder an openness and receptivity to meaning and may even produce defensiveness in the researcher.

Open coding may occur at either a micro or a macro level. Put simply, open coding refers to a process whereby the researcher allows his or herself a free-association *relationship* with the data segment, noting meanings, questioning these meanings, writing memos, planning theoretical samplings and so on. Strauss (1987, p. 63) spoke of open coding as having a 'springboard' function in looking at data. This is because in some ways, the open coding procedure is characterised by a readiness to *jump between* ideas and associations and to remain as open minded as possible about what is being 'seen' in the data.

Theoretical sampling

This term refers to a return to sampling the population and data gathering, that is guided by the emergence of categories or meaning from data already collected. This has a practical impact on the use of grounded theory. What it does, is help support a cycle of data gathering – analysis – then further gathering. It becomes crucial to conduct analysis before further data collection in order that the researcher may be sensitised to issues that may be either present or absent in subsequent work. This presence or absence has the effect of supporting of weakening the emergence of any given category of meaning.

The researcher can therefore be alert to the issue, and can perhaps choose to look at alternative data sources or methods of collection, in order to 'check' or look at the phenomenon from a different angle, as it were. This would be an example of the process of triangulation and the provision of support for a concept from a variety of sources.

Questions of validity and reliability in qualitative research

Reliability is less of an issue than it is in quantitative research, because no claim is being made concerning the replicability of the findings over time. Validity is a concern, however, and is worthy of some discussion here.

As a term, validity comes from the quantitative paradigm and refers to the degree to which a piece of research measures what it purports to measure. In this paradigm, it is one of the conditions that needs to be met in order to be able to infer a causal relationship between two variables (Duffy, 1985). It is argued by some that the concept is alien to the qualitative paradigm (Strauss & Corbin, 1994, p. 266) and that more appropriate indicators of the quality of the research must be found from within the qualitative paradigm itself. Terms such as 'trustworthiness' (Lowenberg, 1993), plausibility or credibility may be preferable.

To some extent, the validity of a developing theory or construction of meaning will depend on the methodology used and the degree to which this is made explicit. Researcher biography is also important. These factors both reveal any potential strengths and weaknesses of the project and place the reader in a sufficiently informed position to be able to evaluate the findings, and make judgements about any connections with other sections of the population if desired or appropriate. This has led to something of an emphasis on 'quality' in qualitative research (Hill-Bailey, 1997). To facilitate this, a readily available and auditable research process for scrutiny by participants and other researchers, needs to be transparent.

Grounded theory's use of a 'constant comparison analysis' (Strauss & Corbin, 1994) has inductive and deductive processes within it. In this sense, a constant verification check is in-built (Miles & Huberman, 1984; Bernard, 1991). It is my experience that the emergence of comparable meaning from different data sets, different samples, and via different methods of data collection, can help to foster a sense of quite elaborate triangulation (Sanders & Liptrot, 1994). The multi-layered 'slices' (Duffy, 1985) of data and related meaning add, I believe, to the quality and trustworthiness of the findings.

Whilst it may be a product of positivistic thinking, I feel it is fair in some ways to ask the question of qualitative research in nursing – 'if a similar study were to be conducted again, would the same findings be made?' I feel that if grounded theory were used, then the answer may well be a hesitant 'yes *and* no'! Reproducing health, social and interpersonal circumstances, dynamics and context in exact detail is likely to be impossible, but differences and inconsistencies between two such hypothetical studies may be able to be explained to some extent. This may be possible for instance, if the studies followed the same general principles and similar conditions in studying the phenomenon under question. 'The same … issues should arise regardless of whether they are conceptualised and integrated a little differently. Whatever discrepancies do arise can usually be explained through re-examination of the data and identification of the alternative conditions that may be operating in each case' (Strauss & Corbin, 1998, p. 267). However, this discussion is inevitably close to a discussion of a form of *reliability* in qualitative research. As such, debate is fraught with difficulties and may in itself be a product of the drift to positivism we are alerted to by Johnson (1999).

Confluence

At this point, it is appropriate for me to integrate this discussion of method in qualitative research with other features of my personal thinking and approach in other spheres of activity as a Consultant Nurse. I have decided to discuss this section under the sub-heading of confluence. I do this because the idea of a joining or a flowing together of influences and practice across my activities is something I have learned to value and see as one way of enhancing the quality and integrity of my work. I have increasingly noted a kind of merging, or integration of ideas that provides me with a – sometimes curious – sense of integration of activities. In essence, this leads me to have the awareness that when I am doing the activity called 'research', I may have some difficulty conceptually separating it from the activities I may call 'psychotherapy, 'mental health nursing' or 'teaching/facilitating'. Each of these activities is concerned with the open exploration of meaning; with the use of self, self-awareness and with a fundamentally collaborative interpersonal style.

To explain this, I would like to set out the principles of approach I endeavour to take into *each* of these activities:

Principle 1: My intention is to collaborate and facilitate, rather than to set myself apart or to 'teach', unless the situation specifically calls for this

Principle 2: I prefer to be open and 'immediate' with my internal experience and reactions to what is going on, and to share this to a level that is appropriate and in keeping. Because of this, I try to view my self as the key tool at my disposal when trying to help or to research

Principle 3: I enjoy feeling free to try new approaches and to be spontaneous, rather than to feel hidebound by prescribed ways of working. I am aware of being at my 'best' when I am aware of, and making some sort of use of, what may be called intuitions

Principle 4: I value learning from others and my experience of working with them. Experiential knowledge is paramount and informs my understanding of theory and research, rather than the reverse

Principle 5: Given the appropriate environmental conditions, people are capable of positive change, substantive understanding and effective problem solving

A related issue is seen in the work of others who have also noted a mutual attraction between mental health nurses and qualitative research. Cutcliffe (2000) suggested that this compatibility could be understood by looking at three significant areas of priority given in the two activities:

1. *The purposeful use of self.* The use of self as the primary research or therapeutic 'instrument' (Lincoln & Guba, 1985) is common to both activities, and is highly prized – being as it is, associated with skill and experience in the field. Qualitative researchers and mental health

nurses are both concerned with the natural processes of everyday life, and the way these processes are understood. The use of self in both fields is concerned with sensitising oneself to ones surroundings in a way that fosters an awareness of its features and dynamics.

2. *The creation of interpersonal relationships*: Both mental health nursing and qualitative research often depend upon the formation of a rapport of some sort with the client or the informant, in order to facilitate the required exploration. Both workers become immersed in the world of the participants, but not so much so that they become lost. An ability to exist in two separate worlds (Cutcliffe, 2000) is required, to allow for a feel for the perspective of the informants, but also to maintain personal integrity and a sense of personal boundary. It is perhaps this skill that allows true helping or enquiry, and helps avoid compulsive rescuing (of clients) or collusion (with informants).

3. *The ability to accept and embrace ambiguity*: The world of both the mental health nurse and the qualitative researcher is made up of uncertainty and ambiguity (Cutcliffe, 2000). There is no expectation of an 'objective truth', and indeed the suggestion that a singular truth has been found will usually receive a cynical response from these workers. Both workers are likely to gravitate to a world of uncertainty, and to feel at ease with this. However, workers in these fields are human, and the avoidance of anxiety may become a powerful impulse on occasions. At these times, the skills of self-awareness function to alert the individual to the urge to achieve closure, early conclusions or forced consensus.

The words of Strauss & Corbin (1994) also add to the debate, when they suggest that the characteristics of a grounded theorist include:

1. the ability to step back and critically analyse situations
2. the ability to recognise the tendency towards bias
3. the ability to think abstractly
4. the ability to be flexible and open to helpful criticism
5. sensitivity to the words and actions of respondents

... which could arguably also be among key descriptors of the effective mental health nurse.

Summary

This chapter has attempted to set out some of the key considerations to be made by the Consultant Nurse when considering research design or when critically reading evidence that they may wish to use to underpin practice. The philosophical, epistemological and methodological bear-traps are many, and the unwary researcher may readily fall into difficulties regarding the coherence or trustworthiness of any work done.

The Consultant Nurse is very likely to be an increasingly crucial figure in the use of research findings, alongside a hopefully increasing profile in the generation of findings that provoke thought, debate and practice development in mental health nursing.

The choices open to the nurse researcher are many and at times, bewildering. Currently, as discussed elsewhere in this text, there is great pressure to adopt positivistic, quantitative methodology as routine when investigating nursing and mental health phenomena. It has not been the purpose of this chapter to criticise this per se. Rather, my intention is to encourage Consultant Nurses to consider the value of structured and rigorous qualitative methods – such as grounded theory – in terms of its compatibility with the essence and core values of mental health nursing itself. A secondary intention is to contribute to redressing the balance of attention given to positivism in current nursing rhetoric.

References

Barker P (1997b) Towards a meta-theory of psychiatric nursing practice *Mental Health Practice* 1(4), pp. 18–21.

Barker P (1997a) The craft of care, collaborative caring in psychiatric nursing. In: Tilley S (ed.) *The Mental Health Nurse*. Routledge, London

Benner P (1984) *From novice to expert: excellence and power in clinical nursing practice*. Adison Wesley, Menlo Park.

Brooker C, Fallon I, Butterworth A, Goldberg D, Graham-Hole V, Hillier V (1994) The outcome of training community psychiatric nurses to deliver psychosocial intervention. *British Journal of Psychiatry*, 165, pp. 222–230.

Burnard P (1991) A method of analysing interview transcripts in qualitative research. *Nurse Education Today*, 11, pp. 461–466.

Burnard P, Hennigan B (2000) Qualitative and quantitative approaches in mental health nursing: moving the debate forward. *Journal of Psychiatric and Mental Health Nursing*, 7(1), pp. 1–6.

Clarke L (1996) Participant observation in a secure unit: care, conflict and control. *Nursing Times Research*, 1(6), pp. 431–440.

Coffey A, Atkinson P (1996) *Making Sense of Qualitative Data*. Sage, London

Coyle J (1999) Exploring the meaning of 'dissatisfaction' with health care: the importance of 'personal identity threat'. *Sociology of Health and Illness*, 21(1), pp. 95–124.

Cutcliffe J (1997) The nature of expert psychiatric nurse practice: a grounded theory study. *Journal of Clinical Nursing*, 6(4) pp. 325–332.

Cutcliffe J (1998) Is psychiatric nursing research barking up the wrong tree? *Nurse Education Today*, 18, pp. 257–258.

Cutcliffe J (2000) Mental health nurses and qualitative research methods: a mutual attraction? *Journal of Advanced Nursing*, 31(3), pp. 590–598.

Dawson PJ (1997) Thoughts of a wet mind in a dry season: the rhetoric and ideology of psychiatric nursing. *Nursing Inquiry*, 4, pp. 69–71.

Denzin NK, Lincoln YS (eds) (1994) Introduction: entering the field of qualitative research. In: *Handbook of Qualitative Research*. Sage, London.

Duffy ME (1985) Designing nursing research: the qualitative-quantitative debate. *Journal of Advanced Nursing*, 10, pp. 225–232.

Geertz C (1973) *The Interpretation of Cultures: Selected Essays*. Basic Books, New York.

Glaser BG, Strauss A (1967) *The Discovery of Grounded Theory*. Aldine, Chicago.

Gournay K, Ritter S (1997) What future for research in mental health nursing? *Journal of Psychiatric and Mental Health Nursing*, 4, pp. 441–446.

Guba EG (1990) *The Paradigm Dialogue*. Sage, London.

Guba EG, Lincoln YS (1998) Competing paradigms in qualitative research. In: *The Landscape of Qualitative Research: Theories and Issues*. Sage, London.

Glaser BG (1978) *Theoretical Sensitivity: Advances in the Method of Grounded Theory*. Sociology Press, California.

Glaser BG (1992) *Emerging vs. Forcing: Basics of Grounded Theory Analysis*. Sociology Press, California.

Hill-Bailey P (1997) Finding your way around qualitative methods in nursing research. *Journal of Advanced Nursing*, 25(1), pp. 18–22.

Jackson S, Stevenson C (1998) The gift of time from the friendly professional. *Nursing Standard*, 12(51), pp. 31–33.

Johnson M (1999) Observations on positivism and pseudoscience in qualitative nursing research. *Journal of Advanced Nursing*, 30(1), pp. 67–73.

Lincoln YS, Guba EG (1985) *Naturalistic Enquiry.* Sage, London.

Lowenberg JS (1993) Interpretive research methodology: broadening the dialogue. *Advances in Nursing Science,* 16(2), pp. 57–69.

Marshall J (1981) Making sense as a personal process. In: Reason P & Rowan J (eds) *Human enquiry: a sourcebook of new paradigm research.* Wiley, London.

McKenna H (1997) Theory construction in nursing: an overview. *Nursing Research,* 23(1), pp. 4–13.

McLeod J (2001) *Qualitative Research in Counselling and Psychotherapy.* Sage, London.

Miles MB, Huberman AM (1994) *Qualitative Data Analysis: a Sourcebook of New Methods.* Sage, London.

Moody LE (1990) *Advancing Nursing Science Through Research.* Sage, California.

Morse JM (1997) *Completing a Qualitative Project, Details and Dialogue.* Sage, London.

Morse JM, Field PA (1995) *Qualitative Research Methods for Health Professionals* (2nd edn). Sage, London.

Pearson A (1992) Knowing nursing: emerging paradigms in nursing. In: Robinson K, Vaughan B (eds), *Knowledge for Nursing Practice.* Butterworth Heinneman, Oxford.

Rosenhan DL (1973) On being sane in insane places. *Science,* 179, pp 250–258.

Sanders P, Liptrott D (1994) *Qualitative Research Methods for Counsellors.* PCCS Books, Manchester.

Simmons S (1995) From paradigm to method in interpretive action research. *Journal of Advanced Nursing,* 21(5), pp. 837–884.

Strauss A (1987) *Qualitative Analysis for Social Scientists.* Cambridge University Press, Cambridge.

Strauss A, Corbin J (1994) Grounded theory methodology. In: Denzin NL, Lincoln YS (eds) *Handbook of Qualitative Research.* Sage, London, pp. 273–285.

Strauss A, Corbin J (1998) *Basics of Qualitative Research: Techniques and Procedures for Developing Grounded Theory,* 2nd edn. Sage, London.

Williams A (1990) Reading feminism in fieldnotes. In: Stanley, L (ed.) *Feminist Praxis: Research Theory and Epistemology in Feminist Sociology.* Routledge, London.

CHAPTER NINE

Cognitive behavioural therapy as a basis for practice development on an acute in-patient unit

Ian Trodden

Introduction

The aim of the chapter is to offer a practical and everyday insight into the functions of the Consultant Nurse's role, and more specifically, to illustrate my own approach to translating these functions into practice. The context of my illustration is an acute in-patient setting within Tees and North East Yorkshire NHS Trust, toward the extreme North of the large patch this Trust covers.

The core role of the Consultant Nurse is to be an 'expert practitioner' and the guidance is that this function should constitute fifty percent of the activity of the role (Department of Health, 1999). I am clear in my mind that we as Consultant Nurses must provide clinical expertise in practice: not to do so would be to risk credibility and potential impact on improving patient care. Here though, by 'clinical expertise', I refer not only to working in isolation with patients and functioning as a clinical nurse specialist. While such practitioners can influence the practice of others, often the impact is limited and the workers tend to work alone (Reed *et al.*, 1998). My interpretation of the concept of clinical expertise involves working very closely with a number of people in the pursuit of developing the way they deliver care, think about and develop their practice. This interpretation requires a mature, collaborative style and a willingness to support others, rather than always going for heroic interventions on one's own.

For my purposes in this chapter, two case illustrations will highlight the mechanism I refer to, in bringing about change in practice and also the different levels of impact that can be made by starting with the patient as the focus of care. (See elsewhere in this text for further discussion on levels of impact.)

I have spoken to a number of colleagues who have expressed concerns that expectations from their organisations have led them to dilute the expert practitioner function to concentrate on other activity. I believe that if Consultant Nurses can get the expert practitioner function right, not only in time-allocated, but in the *way* we deliver this function, then the other functions of leadership, research and development and education will thrive also as a result. To view practice as a discrete entity is a flawed approach, in that when skilled consultant nurses practice they are contributing to the agendas of education, practice development and research (Manley and Dewing, 2002).

To illustrate the levels of impact across a wider context that good practice can bring, I will look at one individual clinical case study and a group case study, for patients suffering from depression. For reasons of confidentiality the clients' names have been changed. I should say that I am accredited with the British Association of Cognitive Behavioural Psychotherapy. As such my "expertise" is in Cognitive Behavioural therapy.

Case study 1 – individual

Bill was referred directly from the multi-disciplinary team (MDT) for Cognitive Behavioural Therapy (CBT) for psychosis. He is a thirty-eight year-old single man diagnosed as suffering from Schizophrenia. He was diagnosed at the age of 18 and since then had had several admissions to the in-patient environment.

I met with the named nurse, Ron, who gave a detailed case presentation. From the outset it was acknowledged that Ron would work closely with Bill and I. The rationale being that he gains further insight into CBT and its application to someone suffering with a psychosis. An objective is to equip him with skills in the assessment and treatment of patients using this approach, which he then could disseminate into the wider ward team.

Bill and I had a series of brief meetings over that week. From this we were able to collaboratively establish what Bill thought were his main problems at that time. The therapeutic purposes in the early sessions were:

- to convey to Bill that his problems were being taken seriously and would be addressed in therapy
- to identify clearly the problems or targeted symptoms presented. In particular, to identify how different problems may interact, for example, the relationship between hearing voices and feeling depressed
- throughout, the aim of therapy was to reduce the distress Bill experienced as a result of his illness.

(Fowler, Garety, and Kuipers, 1995)

He described two main problems, both of which we were able to define in a problem statement and measure using a Likert scale of 0–8 i.e. "this problem upsets me and/or interferes with my normal activities". 0 = Does not; 8 = very severe (Marks *et al.*, 1986).

Problem 1

'I hear voices telling me to carry out evil acts. I feel physically anxious. I think that I may act on them. This causes me to isolate myself'. He rated this as an 'eight' on our scale.

Problem 2

'I get very angry at the voices. I shout at them but think I must be evil to have them. This causes me to feel depressed.' He rated this also as an eight.

Within each problem statement we attempted to identify the way it makes Bill feel physically (Autonomic physiological reaction – A), what he thinks (Cognitions – C) and how he acts (Behaviours – B) as a result (Lang, 1971). This helped Bill gain an early understanding of the inter-relationship of the above process in functional ways, and likewise for staff, family and friends. We also introduced a second A-B-C model. In this case A = activating event, B = belief and C = consequences. Bill described an activating event as someone looking at him when he is worried about the voices he experiences. His belief would be that he could act out as a result of the voice and the consequence for him that it would be true that he is indeed evil and that no one would ever want to know him. Hence a consequence for Bill would be to avoid others when distressed by the voices.

Following the problem statements Bill then discussed possible targets to help him overcome these problems.

Four targets:
1. To be able to reduce the distress I feel that voices cause me
2. To be able to go out and control my anxiety
3. To be able to control my moods better (anger/depression)
4. To not argue so much with my mum as this upsets me and her.

Bill rated the first three targets as being 8 out of 8 (severe difficulty) in terms of his progress in achieving each target regularly without difficulty. He scored problem 4 at 5/8 (definite difficulty) in achieving each target regularly without difficulty.

The importance for Bill to be able to express his problems and then think in terms of goals was fundamental to him believing that he could control some of the above. It was also a powerful experience for Ron, the named nurse, because he was then able to discuss the above in easily digestible terms for the rest of the care team and Bill's immediate family. In addition, the use of measurements was an integral part of the care planning process to assess whether the care delivered was useful or not. If the latter, we could discuss problems and plan solutions to these, the function of the measurement-taking also served to infuse a culture of subjective evidence and ongoing evaluation of quality and effectiveness.

Related to the above, to aid treatment strategies, and also raise staff awareness – we used a number of psychometric tests during Bill's care and treatment. The Brief Psychiatric Rating Scale (BPRS) was used to determine a global assessment of symptoms and focussed around the positive and negative symptoms that Bill had been experiencing. The choice for this measurement is not only the fact it is well validated, but also easy to use in practice. The Health of the Nation Outcome scale (HONOS, 1995) is used as a matter of course within the Care Programme Approach (CPA) in our in-patient environment.

Psychometric testing results

In respect of the positive symptoms Bill was experiencing in relation to his hallucinations we used both the Belief about voices Questionnaire (BAVQ-Chadwick and Birchwood 1995) and the Cognitive Assessment of Voices Interview Schedule (Chadwick, Birchwood and Trower, 1996). The former assessed four areas about the nature of the voices. In relation to Bill his voice was malevolent with no evidence of benevolence. In terms of scoring on resistance Bill scored 9/9 indicative of resistance; on engagement scores he scored 2/8.

The cognitive assessment of voices interview schedule was used to cover the following topics: onset; current experiences of voices (triggers, safety behaviours, content, number of voices and form); feelings and behaviours associated with the voices; beliefs about the voices' source, purpose, omnipotence, compliance and associated negative person evaluations (Chadwick, Birchwood and Trower, 1996).

The above was extremely useful in enabling Bill and the treatment team to get an idiosyncratic view of his experiences of the voice he hears. It was also an invaluable semi-structured interview schedule for the staff to practice in role-plays and then use as part of their assessment skills with some of their patients.

From the above we were able to identify a number of issues. Bill generally heard the voice of a man through his ears that would tell him that everyone hates him, as he is evil. It commands him to harm someone and advises him how to do it. The voice is extremely critical about him and sometimes his mum. It tends to be worse leading up to his monthly depot and if he has not be sleeping or has been in conflict with his mum. The voice frightens, angers and saddens him and he will often isolate himself so that he does not harm anyone. Bill believes the voice is there, as a punishment for him being bad when younger but did not at this stage elaborate further. He resists acting on the commands because he believes he could not be evil yet will also avoid others when voice is very strong. he acknowledged therefore a fear he could act on it as why would he therefore avoid. As stated, the assessment is a very useful way to engage with the patient. However my experience in using this in practice is to be very sensitive when using it as it can elicit a number of powerful emotions. Supervision is key when using these tools.

Other measurements used for negative symptoms were the Schedule for the Assessment of Negative Symptoms (SANS) (Andreasen, 1982). This scale assesses twenty of the negative symptoms: affective flattening, alogia, avolition/apathy, anhedonia/asociality and attention. This with the Social Functioning Scale (SFS, Birchwood, Smith and Cochrane, 1990) highlighted how little time Bill spent in interaction with others. His main source of communication was that of his mum and has been noted at times this caused conflict and distress for both parties. The care plan therefore reflected the need to be sensitive to his negative symptoms whilst encouraging ongoing activities on the ward and a referral to day hospital services. A full occupational assessment further complimented the care planning for treatment of his negative symptoms. The Beck Depression Inventory (Beck and Greer, 1987) also highlighted that Bill was experiencing moderate levels of depression this was indicated by a score of 24 (from possible 60).

Implications of assessment processes and results

As one can see from the above, assessment and level of engagement go hand in hand. It is important to use the assessment tools to go beyond diagnosis into more meaningful formulations. This will enable a collaborative delivery of an evidence-based treatment strategy. The strategy by its very nature needs to be tailored to meet the needs of the patient. It should enhance the nurse's ability to understand the unique meaning and world from which the patient operates, and foster a shared understanding.

During assessment and formulation, the development of a shared understanding is guided by the following principles:

1. Psychotic symptoms become largely understandable once enough information about the person's experience of them has been gathered.
2. Many of the characteristics of psychotic symptoms fluctuate as if on a continuum so that, for instance, levels of conviction in strange, worrying thoughts vary and voices change in volume.
3. All psychotic experience is on a continuum with normal physiological functioning, so that symptoms represent an extreme of normality rather than something that is categorically different.

4. Developing a shared understanding of psychosis is underpinned by knowledge of theoretical models.

(Mills, p. 134, 2000)

Stress vulnerability

Once such theoretical model that Bill and the treatment team focused on was the Stress Vulnerability Model (Zubin and Spring, 1977). The stress vulnerability model proposes that psychosis is by its very nature an episodic problem. The episodes are activated by a number of factors, and that stressful life events interact with vulnerability factors. This can determine whether someone is pushed over the 'psychosis threshold' as it were.

Vulnerability factors include family history of psychosis, poor social support and poor self-care. If some vulnerability factors are present and there are also areas of stress such as bereavement, loss of job and so forth then this may increase someone's vulnerability to illness. The normalisation rationale is not only helpful for patients to understand their illness but guides mental health professionals in their ways of thinking. The important message from the stress vulnerability model is that there are things the person with psychosis can do to help towards reducing vulnerability to symptoms. Furthermore it helps target and plan for possible relapse signatures. In relation to Bill, when stressed his sleep pattern would deteriorate. He would also isolate himself more and participate in less activity. This would lead to more time spent focussing on the distressing voices. As a result, he would become trapped in a vicious circle. Planning services to help with this on discharge was therefore a priority.

Application of the stress-vulnerability model with Bill

By using this approach Bill was able to identify closely with the above. Together, Bill, Ron and myself were able to map the historical evidence behind previous admissions, giving us a detailed analysis of the stresses that had led Bill to become excessively distressed. This historical perspective was then our foundation for anticipating potential future difficulties.

A crucial finding of this exploratory work, was that Bill had many skills and strategies that enabled him to effectively manage a number of aspects of his illness to prevent relapse. This helped Bill maintain a belief that he could have more control over his symptoms than he previously thought, thus supporting his esteem and sense of empowerment. It also enabled the team to be more aware of the 'relapse signatures' pertinent to Bill. This was then planned for in care co-ordination. The consequence of using this model was that Bill, his family and the care team were alerted to the issues that had previously almost automatically meant an admission to the in-patient unit. Importantly for the care team, it also produced a powerful shift in how they viewed the nature of psychosis and how to plan idiosyncratic care plans for treatment and discharge in collaboration with the community services.

Treatment strategies to help manage distressing voices: the behavioural experiment

Bill, Ron and I needed to be aware in dealing with this problem the effects of:

- The distress associated with the belief
- The preoccupation with the belief
- The strength of the belief (conviction)
- The persons responses:
  - Acting as if it's true
  - Looking for things associated with the belief
- The increased tendency to jump to conclusions.

Bill acknowledged that in order to manage some of his fears he tended to isolate himself by avoiding going out. In essence, although understandable due to the conviction of his beliefs, the fears were being maintained and strengthened by his behaviour. In collaboration with Bill and the nursing staff, we designed a number of behavioural experiments in the hope of weakening the effects outlined above. Initially the behavioural experiments were nurse assisted. An example of one of these is outlined in Table 1 in the record sheet for noting behavioural experiments.

The rationale behind the experiments was to test out the notion that what we think and feel are not necessarily facts. In Bill's case, the experiments helped collate ongoing evidence that Bill's voice – whilst distressing – was not as powerful as Bill had previously believed. This perspective

Table 1

Situation	Have run out of milk and need to go to the local shop
Experiment	My way of managing my fears is to avoid going out. If I do go out, I will feel anxious – if I don't plan for this I will have a bad experience
Prediction	I will go to the shop for milk when my anxiety level is below 4 (out of 8) and will distract myself with my Walkman and my new Springsteen CD. If I feel too anxious, I will use the special breathing technique that I learned in relaxation class
Outcome	The trip to the shop was very difficult, but I made it and got my milk! I found the tape music helped me feel some 'good control over the voice in my head
What I learned	That I don't need to avoid situations where people might look at me. People sometimes look at me for no special reason. Other people can't hear the voice in my head.

was further supported by returning to the initial measurements (BAVQ). The experiments were not only helpful for Bill but also Ron, and the other nurses involved in Bill's care. They reflected back that their beliefs about helping patients gain both understanding and control over the power of the voice had been challenged and changed in a positive way.

Bill's case study: conclusion

This case study is important in that it highlights the potential benefit of deploying the expert practice function in a shared and collaborative manner with colleagues. As identified, the outcome for the patient was improved care, with the follow up measurements highlighting longer-term benefits for the patient, as at the time of writing (8 months after Bill's most recent admission to hospital) Bill has not been readmitted. The family involvement in the therapeutic process has also changed the way they think and behave, which has had the effect of taking pressure out of those factors known to increase expressed emotion. Ron and the ward staff have learnt new ways of working and the impact this has on their individual practice will have positive benefits for their patients; ongoing supervision has already identified this. Finally the Consultant Psychiatrists have acknowledged and supported these interventions with their patients.

Case Study 2: group work

The next illustration of the expert practice function and its impact on the in-patient environment that I offer, is working in groups using cognitive behavioural approaches.

On my arrival at the unit, it was clear that there had been little recent activity in terms of therapeutic groups, other than recreational activities. From discussions with the patients and the ward team, we identified the need for a group that would equip patients who were suffering from depression with some skills to enable them to be able to both identify and manage their depression more effectively.

Staff were very keen to be involved, and the initial stages involved a core team up-rating their knowledge and skills in CBT by spending time with myself in seminar and skills based learning sessions. The rationale throughout was that by coaching motivated staff, they could in the future run groups and coach other staff. Importantly the patients would also get a better level of evidence-based care. The manual used to guide the training was Mind Over Mood (Padesky and Greenberger 1994). This manual was is an invaluable tool for the patients and staff alike. The format for sessions was also complemented by the work of Wright, Thase, Beck and Ludgate (1993).

A nurse, a psychology assistant and myself ran the first group. I personally collated all the measurements to determine impact on patient well-being and overall efficacy, the measurements including scores from the BDI, BHS and the BAI. The patients also defined their problems and targets and measured these using Likert-like scales as discussed in Bill's care, above. Eight patients were assessed and screened for suitability from the wards as being likely to be able to benefit from the group experience. A key criterion was that each person had wanted to work in a group setting, and felt able to cope with the potential stresses of the work involved.

Group structure

The group ran over an eight-week period with weekly sessions lasting two hours. The following programme gives an outline indication of the content of each session.

Session 1: Introduction to the cognitive model
- Introduce and discuss diagram of the cognitive model
- Illustrations of linkages between situation, thoughts, feelings and behaviours
- Examples from patient's own experience
- Homework: Read chapter 1 of Mind Over Mood (Padesky and Greenberger 1994).

Session 2: Recognising automatic thoughts
- Review cognitive model
- Review homework
- Definition of automatic thoughts
- Illustrations of automatic thoughts
- Elicit automatic thoughts associated with agenda items
- Homework: Three-column diary of thought record (situation, thoughts, feelings).

Session 3–4: Modifying automatic thoughts
- Review cognitive model, definition of automatic thoughts
- Review homework
- Introduce whole diary of thought record (evidence for/against thought and alternate balanced thought)
- Define and illustrate three methods of changing automatic thoughts
- Work on automatic thoughts associated with agenda items
- Homework: return to thought record and practice developing alternative, functional thoughts.

Session 5: Recognising cognitive errors
- Review cognitive model, automatic thoughts
- Review homework
- List and define thinking errors
- Identify thinking errors associated with agenda items
- Homework: identify own habits in terms of thinking errors.

Session 6: Reaching goals – the step-wise approach
- Review cognitive model; emphasise relationship between cognitive and behaviour

- Review homework
- Introduced graded activity scheduling
- Design graded activity programme
- Homework: use weekly activity schedule.

Session 7: cognitive-behavioural rehearsal

- Review cognitive model, emphasise relationship between cognitions and behaviour
- Review homework
- Describe and illustrate rehearsal techniques
- Perform role-plays and cognitive-behavioural rehearsal with agenda items
- Homework: rehearse strategies (behavioural experiments).

Session 8: review cognitive-behavioural model

- Review homework
- Review previous sessions
- Review measurements
- Discuss blue prints for survival
- Feedback on group experiences
- Homework: Continue to use learned strategies and workbook.

Impact of the group

For the patients in the group the outcomes both in qualitative and quantitative terms were mixed. At the end of the eight sessions four of the original eight in the group had attended all the sessions, with four patients having dropped out. The feedback questionnaire produced a number of reasons as to why this was, with the main themes being that they were being discharged or on extended leave and they found working in groups more difficult than previously expected. These issues and others will be discussed in the "lessons learned" section below. The four who stayed throughout the course gave invaluable feedback. In terms of the pre-group measurements and post-group measurements we can see some encouraging results in Tables 2–4).

The 'pre' to 'post' group change in depression (BDI), hopelessness (BHS) and anxiety (BAI) scores as reported above, suggest a positive

Table 2: Beck depression inventory scores

Patient	Pre-group measures	Post-group measures	Change
1	36	22	−14
2	42	20	−22
3	44	18	−16
4	44	24	−20

Table 3: Beck hopelessness scale scores

Patient	Pre-group measures	Post-group measures	Change
1	18	11	−7
2	20	10	−10
3	20	10	−10
4	20	13	−7

Table 4: Beck anxiety inventory scores

Patient	Pre-group measures	Post-group measures	Change
1	14	8	−4
2	15	10	−5
3	16	9	−7
4	14	9	−5

impact of the group process on well being. Whilst this is very encouraging in terms of crucial issues such as reducing suicide risk, clearly the group was not run on any controlled or empirical basis and so the claims made here must be modest and indicative only. However, the staff team's experience of the group process would support the indicators given here, that this was a positive experience for all concerned.

The evaluation and feedback questionnaires completed by the four completing patients indicted the following themes' helpful aspects:

1. The problems they described were being taken seriously
2. The cognitive framework and workbook (Padesky and Grenberger, 1994) made sense
3. Being able to share their experiences with other members of the group made them feel that they were not alone.

Case study 2: group work – lessons learned

The main lesson learned was that the time frame for the group over a period of eight weeks was too long, as the average stay of patients in our acute in-patient service at this time is three weeks. For some patients, once discharged it can be difficult to return to the unit for a number of reasons, and so continuity beyond this point cannot realistically be guaranteed.

Whilst every effort had been made to make sure that there was a commitment to the group as part of the prescribed care package, in reality pressure on beds came before the needs of the group. This fact helps explain the discharges and leave status for some patients, and the consequent fall-out of members of the group. As a result of this, the ward team and the patients decided that the best format for the next group would be for they're to be two sessions per week over a three-week period.

An important lesson learned was that there are nursing staff that are extremely motivated to be involved in the educational component of the training and the therapy process in vivo. It seems to me that the investment in this area has not only made an impact in terms of group work but on the wider therapeutic milieu within the ward, work for the future would include capturing evidence for this observation. Staff seem to me more willing and ready to use the skills and knowledge learned, and to transfer these to their individual clients. We now have a strong cohort of staff that can work as both therapists and co-therapists (with close supervision) using the cognitive model. Groups to date include working with patients who are suffering from depression, anxiety, and anger.

Discussion and conclusion

The two case studies detailed offer an insight into my approach to the fulfilment of the expert practice function of the Consultant Nurse role. As I said at the start, my belief if that through this function, it is possible to deliver the other three functions of:

- leadership
- research and development
- education

... in an integrated fashion *within* the vehicle of practice development and enhancement.

There are of course many other activities outside the case studies, which constitute my personal contribution to practice development in the broadest sense. Among these are regular 'enhanced skills' teaching sessions that I run, which are designed to support staff development and morale – as they feel more and more confident in their ability to deliver purposeful interventions with their patients.

I have also explained that my area of expertise is in CBT, but of course I am a nurse and take great pains to embrace this skills base into this fundamental identity. However, I believe that CBT is an extremely valuable model – not just because of the ever-increasing evidence base regarding its effectiveness, but also because it allows for a readily understandable framework for patients and nurses alike to operate within. This framework of understanding does, I believe, help confer a sense of understanding, purpose, control and composure to both the patient and the nurse. This position is not supportive of anxiety and uncertainty – two of the greatest enemies perhaps, both of mental health, and of purposeful therapeutic activity in the nurse.

References

Chadwick P, Birchwood M (1994) The cognitive assessment of voices schedule. In: Chadwick P, Birchwood M, Trower P (eds) (1996) *Cognitive Therapy for Hallucinations, Delusions and Paranoia*. Wiley, Chichester, pp. 195–200.

Chadwick P, Birchwood M (1995) The beliefs about voices questionnaire. In: Chadwick P, Birchwood M, Trower P (eds) (1996) *Cognitive Therapy for Hallucinations, Delusions and Paranoia*. Wiley, Chichester, pp. 201–202.

Chadwick P, Birchwood M, Trower P (eds) (1996) *Cognitive Therapy for Hallucinations, Delusions and Paranoia*. Wiley, Chichester.

Fowler P, Garety P, Kuipers L (1995) *Cognitive Behaviour Therapy for Psychosis, a Clinical Handbook*. Wiley, Chichester.

Gamble C, Brennan G (2000) *Working with Serious Mental Illness, A Manual for Clinical Practice*. Bailliere Tindall.

Greenberger D & Padesky CA (1995) *Mind Over Mood: Change How You Feel by Changing the Way You Think*. New York: Guilford Press. (First published as *Mind Over Mood: A Cognitive Therapy Treatment Manual For Clients*.)

Marks IM (1986) *The Maudsley Handbook of Behavioural Psychotherapy*. Croom Helm, London.

Mills J (2000) Dealing with voices and strange thoughts. In: Gamble, C & Brennan, G (eds) *Working with Serious Mental Illness, A Manual for Clinical Practice*.

Wright JH, Thase ME, Beck AT & Ludgate JW (eds) (1993). *Cognitive Therapy with Inpatients: Developing a Cognitive Milieu*. New York: Guildford Press.

Zubin J, Spring B (1977) Vulnerability: a new view of schizophrenia. *Journal of Abnormal Psychology*, 86, 260–266.

CHAPTER TEN

Engagement and abstraction

A model for considering the impact of the clinical work of the Consultant Nurse

Gary Wilshaw

Introduction

If the role of the Consultant Nurse is to be truly and significantly 'new', if it is to characterised by 'expert clinical practice' and if it is to meet the two key aspirations expressed in the Health Service Circular *Making a Difference* (1999):

- the provision of better patient outcomes through improvements in the quality of care
- the strengthening of leadership

… then a broad and abstract interpretation of the *spirit* of the role is needed. Elsewhere in this book, it is suggested that when attempting to develop itself, nursing has a propensity to create new roles that mimic the way doctors have divided their own labour, and a tendency to carve up human suffering into a discrete taxonomy that claims to represent the human experience we used to call 'madness'. This is reductionist in its effect, and is partially rooted in the task orientation culture of nursing which remains in existence.

I believe it is important at this time to be able to conceive of the Consultant Nurse's work in ways that are appropriately holistic, non-mechanical and non-fragmentary. An expansive perspective can open up new ways of working that maximise the potential of this new role and its impact on the systems of health care. The model I will describe here provides for a framework within which *all* the work of the consultant nurse may be formulated, considered and evaluated. It is based on the premise that the role is one that is concerned *solely* with care delivery, and allows for a range of apparently subsidiary activities to be directly related to this essential purpose.

Whilst providing boundaries to thoughts about the role of the consultant nurse, the model is also liberating, allowing incumbents to move across systems of care, professional boundaries and among partnership agencies, to push back the barriers to caring responses.

Impact

Appointees to the post of Consultant Nurse are expected to be appropriately senior, authoritative and experienced, to be able to rise to the highest aspirations of the post as hinted at in publications from the Department of Health. Essentially, suggestions abounded that the post ought to be thought of as in many ways equivalent to the medic's Consultant post, with concomitant status both in the care of the service user and in the organisational power structure.

In reality, appointing appropriately experienced, educated and skilled nurses has been less than straightforward. There would appear to be a shortage of such people ready to step into the role, and instead, organisations have had to be ready to appoint people who show the right potential. This is not necessarily a problem in its own right, but needs to be considered in the context of organisational readiness to both support and then to exploit the role in the most imaginative and constructive way possible.

Abstraction

Figure 10.1 represents a model to assist the assessment of the degree to which the Consultant Nurse role is operating across a wide range of activity – from the relatively 'concrete' 1:1 or group clinical activity, through to more 'abstract' health-economy development related activity of a Consultant Nurse 'authorised' to represent the locality and negotiate on its behalf.

To illustrate this model further I will give brief examples of work activity across the scale, moving from the relatively concrete to the sort of work that is more concerned with systemic issues of organisational

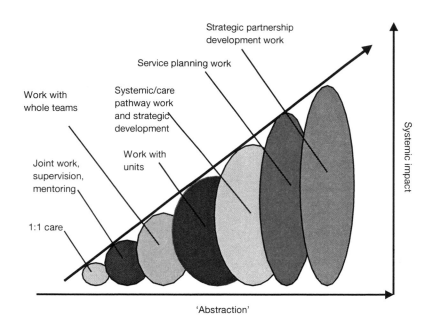

Strategic partnership
development work

Service planning work

Work with
whole teams

Systemic/care
pathway work
and strategic
development

Joint work,
supervision,
mentoring

Work with
units

1:1 care

Systemic impact

'Abstraction'

Figure 10.1

culture, effectiveness and development. I would argue that each of the exemplar activities are legitimate spheres of work for the Consultant and moreover, that the degree to which the post holder may be effective in these areas, is in part dependent upon the ability to *inform* that work with core elements of learning brought from the less-abstract activity lower on the scale. I will discuss the latter point further in a little while, for now though – here are some examples of activity moving up the scale of abstraction.

Example 1: 1:1 care

June, a 22-year-old woman, is referred by her GP. She is depressed, anxious and sleeps only after heavy self-medicating with alcohol. She sometimes has ideas about taking her life.

During assessment, it emerges that June is lesbian and has kept this secret from family and all friends but one. This one close friend had recently been killed in a road accident. In addition to the trauma of the loss of a dear friend, June also lost an important source of support in her attempts to embrace (or perhaps 'deny') her sexuality and personal identity.

During brief integrative psychotherapy, I assisted June to explore her feelings about both her bereavement and her sexuality, and develop plans for the future integration of her more complete identity. After ten contacts, initially set (modest) goals had been met, and agreement to end therapy was reached.

Example 2: Joint work, supervision and mentoring

Mark is a 30-year- old man, referred to the CMHT by probation workers in respect of his aggression and use of violence related to his long-standing personality problems and depression. He has an extensive petty crime record and is in danger of committing more serious violent crime, as his frustrations with life seem to grow.

Mary, his social worker, has become aware that Mark was sexually abused during his time in foster care as a child. She suspects that this experience is important in explaining his current tendency towards aggression. Mary is aware of my own research and practice interests in working with adult survivors of childhood sexual abuse, and had seen a paper I had published on the topic (Wilshaw, 1999).

May and I agreed to meet regularly for the purpose of my supervising her work with Mark and helping her develop the care plan – taking into account the impact of his earlier abuse on his personality structure. We used ideas from Cognitive Analytic Therapy (CAT) to construct a simple formulation that helped to explain much of Mark's behaviour.

Example 3: Work with whole teams

A team of professionals working in a busy A & E department in a large District General Hospital was invited to a seminar looking at ways of responding to those people who present with deliberate self harm.

During the seminar, a Consultant Nurse colleague agreed to a further series of workshops aimed at exploring the use of brief, solution focused techniques during assessment on presentation. Over a period of months, my colleague helped the A & E staff to develop their understanding and modify their practices. Changes made were based on the following ideas:

- That the current presentation can be seen as a valuable opportunity to form a link with the individual, to throw a 'therapeutic lifeline'
- That the presentation can be an opportunity to screen for unde-tected/untreated mental health problems
- That there may be a unique opportunity to begin a conversation that validates experience of suffering, identifies strengths and resources that have helped the person cope thus far after Talmon (1990).

After a time, the work was evaluated in terms of impact on patient care and staff confidence in responding to those presenting in this way. Paper-work supporting the assessment process was modified to be solution-focused in nature and the initiative was publicised at local conferences.

Example 4: Work with units

A unit of two acute in-patient wards was interested in being supported to take regular time-out to reflect on their practice. I agreed to facilitate weekly meetings of an hour at a fixed time and venue. The team members who attended were mainly nurses and occupational therapists.

Over a period of four months, the teams became increasingly aware that woven into their thoughts were certain small but important obstacles to their *feeling good* about what they did. The factors seemed to frustrate efforts to work effectively, collaboratively and deliver what they consid-ered to be the best help they possibly could give. In particular, factors identified seemed to have the impact of creating a sense of *powerlessness* over control of the very environment that they worked and engaged patients within – such as the authority to refuse to admit a heavily intox-icated patient when the unit policy was that this would not occur.

Through a process of assisting the teams to articulate and analyse their feelings, a series of issues were clarified. These issues represented key frus-trations and dynamics that they felt undermined their ability to provide best care. After some time, the unit leader made an assertive bid to pres-ent these issues at the most senior management forum, along with sug-gested solutions and other plans to enhance the coherence of care planning across professional groups. The teams presented their ideas and were supported in making important changes in policy and practice.

Example 5: Systemic/care pathway work and strategic development

Mental health problems in the perinatal period are common, but not always detected at an early stage (Oates, 2000). With this in mind, a dialogue was opened with maternity services managers to discuss current practice and to identify areas for development.

I accepted a commission to identify an appropriate method of screening, to detect mental health problems (or their predictors) in the antenatal period. In addition, I worked with colleagues to devise care pathways and to promote positive responses to mental health problems midwives and health-visitors might detect in the perinatal period.

A literature review was conducted and a tool identified that appeared suitable in terms of its validity, reliability and practicality. Contact with the American authors responsible for the tool was established, and permission was obtained to both modify and use the tool as part of an action research project. The tool was examined by a research group of primary care mental health colleagues, midwives and health visitors. A research design and protocol was then agreed with colleagues, ethical permission was obtained, and testing of the tool commenced at the 'booking-in' stage (14 weeks) and the subsequent 32-week stage of gestation.

The research team met regularly as screening progressed, to review the tool's usefulness and all other aspects of the research design. Simultaneously, the care pathways that were put into place were also monitored and discussed as and when they were actioned. Concerns and findings that the screening brought to light were reviewed at these meetings, and decisions made regarding appropriate courses of action.

The whole process was recorded, all data was shared among the team, relevant managers and other interested parties in the locality. Out of a sample of forty pregnant women, ten were assessed as having previously undetected mental health concerns, and were provided with an appropriate response. The responses included a fast-tracking to primary care mental health workers (PCMHW), or care from the woman's midwife that was supported by the PCMHW.

The research team has presented the work at several local and national conferences, and is in the process of writing a paper for publication on the work, and sharing ideas at seminars in the locality. The work has also attracted attention in neighbouring counties, with professionals from these areas networking across in order to inform their own plans for related projects.

Example 6: Service Planning work

A 'key deliverable' in mental health service developments at the time of writing is the development of a Crisis Response & Resolution (CR&R) facility. The introduction of this in the area in which I work has been embraced positively and imaginatively. A team of well-motivated, experienced and skilled people were recruited and immediately engaged in the development of an operational policy and so on.

The locality director, general managers, associate medical director and myself convened stakeholder workshops to consider the impact of this new service on the 'shape' of the entire system – given that a key intention was to impact directly on factors such as admission rates to the acute unit and the nature of work undertaken by CMHTs.

A model of the new system was developed and agreed by consensus at these workshops, based around the CR&R functioning as a single entry point for referrals. At this point, my role became that of contributing to the leadership of a change process that had implications for almost everyone involved in mental health services locally.

Work after this point included the development of better practices in the maintenance an SMI (Serious Mental Illness) register by the CMHT in collaboration with primary care; streamlining of care-planning/review and dialogue between teams and three consultant psychiatrists; and better focus on processes of *disengagement* with patients once needs had been met. As can be seen in these examples, many of the work-streams at this point had the dual and complementary elements of systemic capacity building and 'purposeful' engagement with people in relation to the needs.

Example 7: Strategic partnership development work

In my own locality, the post I occupy has been embraced into the most senior management group and its functions. There are many examples of being fully involved and integrated in planning and decision making (included becoming a member of the most senior management forum) that influence the overall direction of developments in the local 'health care economy'. I use this term because it points to the broad landscape of organisations, functions and people that have an influence in shaping those factors impacting on the mental well-being of a community.

Mental health is clearly not about hospitals or care teams. It is more importantly related to matters of employment, schooling, poverty, a sense community, housing, child care, family ... and so on. Services claim to address mental *health*, but often merely address mental *illness*. It is not my purpose to review these issues here, but to acknowledge that an organisation interested in impacting on mental health will concern itself with this mercurial economy, and the factors that shape it.

An example of strategic partnership development work I would offer here is an on-going project where my post is deployed in a way that represents the Trust I work for, in the context of a broad, multi-agency initiative to address a healthcare economy issue very relevant to mental health.

Monies were secured by the Primary Care Trust (PCT) to develop a service to better meet the needs of the homeless population of a seaside town. Over a period of eighteen months, I represented the mental health Trust in planning meetings that spent the monies on Health Visiting, Nurse Practitioner, General Practitioner and Primary Care Mental Health Worker facility. In addition to spending the money, hard negotiations took place to initiate new routes to care for this population and at the time of writing, efforts are under way to integrate care 'into the mainstream', in order to avoid the creation of a 'ghetto'.

Systemic impact

This component of the framework is a direct reflection of the level of abstraction scale. That is to say, the further up the level of abstraction scale a care delivery 'act' is, the greater the is potential for a far reaching and systemic impact.

If we take the seven examples of acts of care above, it can be seen that example six, for instance has the *potential* to influence the quality of care delivery across a broad area – e.g. the entire locality. The acts of care at the lower level of abstraction (e.g. one), will arguably influence June's life only – or at best of course, that of June and her friends/family. Example three concerns work that is clearly designed to impact on the care being given to those who present in A & E with deliberate self-harm. Here however, the Consultant Nurse is able to work alongside others and contribute to developmental processes that may impact not just on this patient group, but also on other work done by these people in that specific care setting or beyond.

In example six, it can be seen that the staff involved planning this service development, are likely to develop their skills and thinking concerning mental health, collaborative work, care pathways, data analysis, using assessment tools and so on. In addition to the care of people in Crisis, the likelihood is that the staff concerned will take this learning and apply it elsewhere. Clearly, there would be value in evaluating the empirical reality behind my supposition.

It can be seen that there is a trade-off between the 'impact' or value of the act of care, between the 'system' and the individual person in care. The higher up the level of abstraction is the act of care delivery, the greater the potential impact the Consultant Nurse may have on the whole system or the local healthcare organisations. At the same time, the *direct* impact upon the person by the Consultant Nurse is reduced.

Role and functional coherence: facilitating learning across the whole system

A final and important dynamic in this way of thinking about the role of the consultant nurse requires a question to be asked. That question is 'how do these apparently discrete areas of activity (exemplified above) relate to each other?

The answer I think is represented in Figure 10.2. The Consultant Nurse has perhaps what is a unique opportunity, to convey *cultural intelligence* from one part of the system to the next. The impact of this is to promote coherence, or at least to draw attention to *incoherence* where this is present.

If we look specifically at the core material learned at one level of activity, it is not difficult to name what it might be. The clinical 'root' work of the consultant nurse enables a grounding in the realities of suffering, and what it is like to seek help. This 'client centredness' can thus be carried into all other work further along the abstraction scale, and deployed

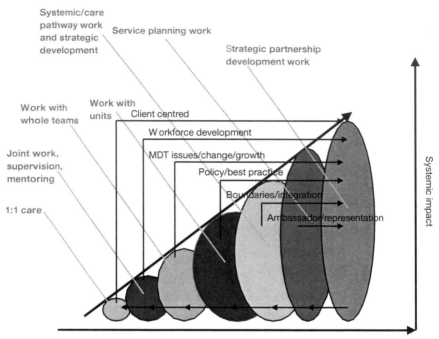

Figure 10.2

at all points where this perspective is crucial. From supervisory work and work with teams/units, the consultant learns about issues of skills that remain under-utilised (or under developed) and about the way teams work/do not work. From strategic development and service planning work, the consultant develops a better understanding of cross-agency collaboration and blocks to so-called 'seamless' care, and so on. The direction of travel of this 'cultural intelligence' is not one-way. The post-holder also is able to take broader, systemic understanding of strategic issues – directly into work with teams and indeed direct care with patients.

My feeling is that it is almost as if there is a key role to be played in enabling the unearthing and movement of this 'cultural intelligence' around the system in the way I describe. Managers and other workers do this of course, but there is something unique in the fact that the basis of the activity is direct involvement in the care of those people in need.

Discussion and implications for practice

I have set out a rudimentary framework that may assist Consultant Nurses, and perhaps other workers, to conceptualise their work in terms of its relevance to care practices in the broadest sense. My rationale for this being an important process, rests on my assertion that *all* activity of the Consultant Nurse needs to be anchored in terms of 'clinical impact', if the role is to be exploited to its potential. The framework may be used in at least two distinct ways.

Professional self-monitoring

Firstly, as a part of a process of self-monitoring, it may be of value for the Consultant Nurse to regularly audit the work they do, plotting activities on the abstraction scale as exemplified in this chapter. In doing this, a picture should emerge of the *spread* across the scale that the various activities represent. If there can be an 'ideal' picture, I would argue it would suggest involvement in work across the spectrum of abstraction. This should signal a blend of 'hands on' work with patients, and a range of other activities concerning influence on a broader scale across the health care agencies. A not incidental further value of this reflection of work done, is that it allows for a close integration and acute awareness of clinical issues, with the processes of strategic thinking and care systems development. In my own case, I am often aware that my thinking on most tasks, is guided by my recent experience with patients, patient groups and their families. This in-built awareness may prove to be a key strength of the role and may provide a function of clinical intelligence in leadership functions.

The second key use of this scale follows on from the first. If, after auditing the work engaged in as described above, there are 'gaps' or parts of the scale of abstraction that are under-represented, then the Consultant Nurse may chose to respond. The tool is of use primarily to raise the awareness of the Consultant. At best it is a tool to support professional awareness and aid decision-making about the sort of projects and activities that out to be set-up or selected, when prioritising work.

This function may assist in the development of the *role*, not just the *person* in the role. It is perhaps important at this early stage in the establishment of Consultant Nurse posts, that the greatest possible impact value is developed – which will require post holders to avoid remaining in personal 'comfort zones', and engaging in work that is familiar, tried and tested – and perhaps simply brought brought from previously held posts.

Conclusions

The Consultant Nurse posts offers great promise in terms of the quality of care available and access of those in need to that care. For this promise to be realised, incumbents and services alike must examine the range, scope and quality of the work being engaged in to ensure a broad and systemic impact. It is not enough for the Consultant Nurse to deliver expert practice to specific patients, families or small groups. The impact of the role ought to be felt across local whole-systems of care, if this role is to be truly distinct, and if it is to offer the sort of clinical leadership that will make a difference to people's lives.

References

Oates, M. (2000) *Perinatal Mental Health Services*. Royal College of Psychiatrists, London.

Talmon, M. (1990) *Single Session Therapy*. Jossey-Bass: San Francisco.

Wilshaw, G. (1999) Perspectives on surviving childhood sexual abuse. *Journal of Advanced Nursing*, 30(2), pp. 303–309.

CHAPTER ELEVEN

Moving beyond a support act

Clinical supervision and the Consultant Nurse role

Steve Harrison

Introduction

Clinical supervision in the mental health nursing arena offers exiting opportunities to develop the immense talents of nurses. The process has however, struggled to establish itself in a culture that is not always conducive to the growth and maturation that such activities require. The development of the Consultant Nurse role heralds a shift in attitudes, which can help the values of reflective practice mature and become more fruitful for all concerned. Let us explore the issues in greater detail.

There is a reasonable chance that I, or a close member of my family, will at some stage of their life need the services of mental health nurses. The unfortunate nurse who aspires to influence for the better the mental health of my family or myself need to first of all convince me of the following:

1. Do they know what they are doing?
2. Do they methodically think about what they are doing?
3. Do they rigorously question their thinking about this process?

I like to delude myself, that even though I may be in the throes of a depressive illness, when I meet my key nurse I will fix them with a steely glare and cheerfully fire these questions at him or her.

Of course what I'm really asking is,' 'Do you have regular, good quality clinical supervision?' I suspect that if I'm admitted to a mental health unit tomorrow I would be much more likely to hear 'sort of', 'when there's time' or even 'you're joking' as an answer rather than 'of course, now please get out of bed!'. When thought about in these straightforward terms, clinical supervision seems to be a clear-cut commonsense proposition. Why then, does clinical supervision seem to be such a slippery and elusive feature of professional practice to institute? What steps can be taken to support this process? Finally, what contribution can the Consultant Nurse make to the development of reflective practice in the mental health arena?

I think a key issue in addressing the elusive quality of supervision lies in the meanings attached to 'supervision'.

Meanings of supervision

There is an academic game that I could play at this stage. I find a rudimentary definition for 'supervision', pretend to have a think about it, pronounce it unworthy and then produce a more sophisticated version from up my sleeve that comes up to my high standards.

On this occasion I don't think I'll bother if it's all right with you, as there is already enough confusion about the meaning of supervision without my little indulgence. Instead let us adopt an accepted definition and then consider the existing multitude of activities that come under the heading 'supervision'.

Perhaps one of the most cited authors on the subject who fits in the context of nursing frameworks is Christopher Johns (1993) He defines clinical supervision as:

> 'an intensive, interpersonally focused, one-to-one relationship in which one person is designed to facilitate the development of therapeutic competence in the other person.'

This definition is concise, practical and clear. It serves its purpose well. Having chosen a 'good enough' definition, what of the many actions that go under the banner of supervision?

Castledine (1994) noted succinctly that supervision meant different things to different people. The comparisons made by Castledine are between supervision as a means of ensuring that a number of tasks get done, and supervision which focuses on ensuring work is up to a set standard, for example, making certain that an assignment is up to the right academic requirements. Working in a multi-disciplinary mental health team it is clear that this is only one potential comparison. In social work, a supervision session is traditionally a time when a manager checks all the social worker's case load to ensure practice is safe and effective. It is primarily a management tool.

By contrast, medical colleagues use supervision as a training arena for junior staff. The focus seems to be upon applying knowledge to practice. Cutcliffe and Proctor (1998) emphasise that supervision in nursing is concerned with reflecting upon practice, increasing awareness both of oneself and of solutions to clinical problems.

From a supervised person's perspective, one could find oneself on the receiving end of management scrutiny, structured teaching or an adaptation of a counselling situation depending upon which professional group you were allied to. These different viewpoints carry with them different implications for participants. Goorapah (1996) identifies that control could over-shadow staff development as a central theme of the process. It is further suggested here that although an individual's learning may be a central theme, the experience of supervision could be construed as punitive and intrusive. This could be the case if the clinician being supervised lacks a robust sense of their own self worth, and the supervisor does not possess the range of interpersonal skills required of an effective facilitator.

If we pluck up our courage and adopt the principle that Carl Rogers (1967) suggested, that awareness of the facts, no matter how unpalatable, is 'friendly'. The first fact that we can get acquainted with is that our starting point (the meanings of supervision) is far from clear-cut. Luckily, the task that has been given to me dictates that I focus upon a nursing frame of reference.

It's good to talk

In 1999 lecturers at the University of York used (CiNAHL) to review the nursing literature regarding Clinical Supervision. Four hundred and sixty three articles were published. Only eleven could be construed as research. Of these only Tony Butterworth's (1997) study 'It is Good to Talk' was both of a substantial size and conducted in the U.K. The key messages arising from this study were that supervision was perceived to be a beneficial process on a number of levels for participants. It was, however, difficult to link this to positive outcomes for patients.

A significant and substantial piece of work came from Scandinavia, conducted by Hyrkas, Koivula and Paunonen (1999). This work established the state of research and key issues surrounding clinical supervision in a nursing context. Their view was that developmentally, the phenomenon was in its infancy, and that there was insufficient evidence to demonstrate that clinical supervision was a reliably effective process. It is noted here that there are differences in the British tradition of viewing supervision as being synonymous with mentorship and preceptorship. By contrast the Scandinavian model focuses more on post qualification professional development. Commonly cited authors elsewhere have similar messages.

Fowler (1996) notes a lack of structure or theoretical grounding beneath the general claim that supervision is a valuable use of clinical resources. Wolsey and Leach (1997) once again point out that the question of clinical outcomes has not been tackled to any significant extent. It seems therefore, that even in a nursing context the meanings underlying the term 'clinical supervision' are hard to grasp, both in terms of theoretical grounding and effectiveness. But just because it is a difficult puzzle to unravel does that mean it isn't worth the effort? There are in my view, enough indicators to suggest that the aspirations of clinical supervision are goals worth pursuing further at this stage.

First principles

What do we know so far? Clinical supervision has many meanings, even in a nursing context uncertainties exist, particularly in regard to a theoretical foundation for the process, and a lack of evidence concerning improved patient outcomes. Nevertheless, Butterworth's (1997) study showed some signs for optimism, and reminded us that the process is in a formative stage. It is logical to reflect, therefore, that if we are dealing with a process in its infancy, we should, like any good parent, have appropriate expectations, and be patient with teething troubles.

What would we appropriately consider to be the core tasks of supervision? Proctor (1986) gives us a useful and established framework to gather our thoughts. The functions outlined here are as follows: the formative aspects of supervision, that is to say, the development of competence. The normative aspects, which relate to professional and organisational standards, and finally, the restorative qualities of supervision, which is, in essence, concerned with supporting clinicians. Let us look at support first.

Support

Perhaps the most consistently cited feature of clinical supervision in relationship to nursing is that of a means of providing support to clinicians working in a challenging environment. Hawkins and Shohet (1994) emphasise the importance of supervision as a means of creating a support system. Dexter and Wash (1995) identify patchy supervision mechanisms that render clinicians and their clients under supported. Finally, Proctor (1986) sees the restorative quality of supervision as a key aspect of any reflective practice.

It is hard to argue against the notion that nurses work in a highly challenging environment and face numerous stresses which could be debilitating if not countered. There could, however, be limitations on an activity that primarily concerned itself with supportive interventions. Heron (1990) cites many ways in which this particular activity can degenerate if unaccompanied by interventions with other intentions – such as catharsis for instance. Support delivered indiscriminately can be patronising, collusive or worse-validating inappropriate practice.

There is clearly a balance to achieve between establishing a sense of support and not being suffocating or sustaining situations that are ripe for a challenge.

Challenge

What of the formative aspirations of supervision? If supervision aims to increase the expertise of clinicians surely there is a place for challenging practice. This theme is generally not so easily detected but it is, I believe, at the core of the process.

The published material on this theme is less evident than that centring on support. Fisher (1996, pp 443–444) makes the point that supervision is about support as opposed to managerial monitoring. But closer examination reveals that supervision can be, at least in part, driven by challenges, 'what factors influenced your decisions? ... what other choices did you have? ... what other skills do you have to develop?... what have you learned from this experience?' – these are clearly all challenging questions.

It should be noted that throughout Fisher's article the concept of challenging in supervision is not touched upon, but the principles clearly fit. Egan (1994 p. 164) asserts that challenging is a key part of helping people by 'using their ability to construct reality, helping them reconstruct their views of themselves and their worlds in more self enhancing ways'. It seems then that beneath the surface there is a more subtle but valuable dynamic at play. This notion of reconstruction as an enabling action is reinforced by Mezirow (1981 pp. 3–24) who described 'transformation perspective' as the acquisition of knowledge which leads to a change of outlook both on situations and upon the power that people have to influence them. This seems to match with the data and makes sense with the idea of supervision as a vehicle for challenging the ways clinicians construct their professional world.

Challenge to the person

If we accept that there is a process of questioning methods then it logically follows that there is an indirect challenge to the cognitive and emotional processes behind those methods. In other words not only are the professional aspects of supervised nurses under the spotlight but also their personal qualities.

The message here is that through reflection upon action one can arrive at a more personal domain where the *supervisee* becomes the focus and not the immediate clinical problem. Snowball *et al.* (1994 p. 1235) cited the work of Schon (1987) in regard to this complex notion. It is suggested here that reflection is most sought after when overwhelmed, stuck or dissatisfied with performance; therefore discomfort and a degree of emotionally charged material is inextricably linked to the reflective process. The article goes on to discuss the 'reflective practicum ...the virtual world' set in a relatively low-risk environment designed to explore practice. This metaphor is revealing, not a virtual classroom, study, nor consulting area, but an all-encompassing environment where the full spectrum of experience is there to be reconstructed.

Challenging and moving on

Uncertainties, fear of not achieving either self-imposed expectations or the expectations of others, are weighty areas for a supervised nurse to reflect upon. In addition to this, the implication is that the supervisor's challenge is to invite them to move beyond these situations, not merely to reflect or reassure.

Barker (1992, pp. 65–79) argues that a process which exposes the inner aspects of people to scrutiny is 'a potential emotional minefield'. The suggestion is that supervision is a process that not only clarifies options, but also requires the nurse to ask whether he or she is ready to choose how to develop further. This is certainly a challenging notion. Once again, as in the supportive aspects of supervision, key skills are required to challenge constructively, in a supportive and ethical way that does not result in supervised nurses feeling punished or inappropriately scrutinised.

Broader contexts and protective mechanisms

Finally, let us consider the goal of organisational and professional standards. To their credit, several influential frameworks urge supervisors to consider practice in the context of organisational expectations, legal requirements and professional guidelines. This would seem to be a straight-forward task until you consider the scale of organisational expectations, the many ambiguities and contradictions in the law and the broad brush commandments that occasionally find their way into professional guidelines.

The effective supervisor is to some extent concerned with re-examining practice not only for learning and support, nor only considering new action and perspectives. He or she is also concerned with reflection upon the notion of doing or not doing harm to patients by taking action which is disempowering or even directly harmful. Barker (1992 p. 67) saw this as a critical element of supervision – 'Supervision in psychiatric nursing has two main aims: to protect people in care from nurses and to protect nurses from themselves…'. Although the statement appears direct, it alludes to a somewhat intangible problem. That of a nurse locked into their own beliefs about what is best for the patient, which may at times fly in the face of external expectations and changes in practice.

This theme is supported by Goorapah (1997 p. 177) who asserts that supervision had a key role to play in providing an organised vehicle where strengths and weaknesses can be examined in a way that promotes authentic reflection. However, reservations are expressed as to whether a supervisor can overlook his or her ethical responsibility for monitoring standards. It could be argued that the fact that a supervised nurse is assessing interventions to see whether they are sound is inherently ethical. Therefore, by considering options that may be unacceptable in the relative safety of supervision, he is both developing insights into his own abilities, and ensuring that actions have not only been re-examined by him but also by another clinician. Both supervisor and supervised nurse will bring their own contribution to patient care.

A position suggested by Goorapah's work is that when a supervised nurse considers care which to the supervisor may result in adverse consequences, then the supervisor has responsibilities and has to accept that 'supervision may need to be used in a punitive way' (1997 p. 177). In fairness to the author, he is suggesting this when the competence of the nurse is in question. Nevertheless, it could be argued that this position, though ethically strong, is a reductive view of supervision. Jones (1997 p. 1034) makes this point, acknowledging the subtleties inherent in relationships.

> The ambiguity of human experience calls for tentative hypotheses as opposed to a search for absolute truths. It is additionally important that the nurse shares a belief in the theoretical suppositions. We carry out supervision *with* a worker not on them.

This view of supervision as a collaborative arena for dealing with tentative notions, curiosity and possibilities within safe parameters seems to make sense.

Effective supervision, even when considered in a rather basic framework seems to be a complex business. There are clearly many opportunities for a nurse to develop his or her knowledge skills and attitudes as well as using past experiences more thoroughly as a medium for learning.

Restrictive versus developmental supervision

A skilled supervisor, in my view, needs something more than the ability to tackle the core functions of supervision in a methodical way using an established model. A high order skill is to retain the awareness that such models are simply that – 'models'. By all means provide structure to supervision sessions and utilise appropriate frameworks to ensure that participants get a sense of direction and containment, however, supervisors need to apply ideas in a way that is responsive, authentic and not mechanistic. Hawkins and Shohet (1989) draw parallels between supervision and creative play, describing a climate where spontaneity and creativity can emerge. If you were unfortunate enough to be supervising me you would be hard pressed to receive a creative response if you were slavishly following a framework regardless of the ideas I was trying to express. Nurses in my experience can spot 'empathy by numbers' without too much trouble.

Having examined clinical supervision both in terms of its development and also in terms of its stated aims and functions it all seems a bit weighty and daunting. What does strike me as interesting is perhaps the naïve expectation held in some quarters that this process was ever going to be a neat linear journey: one that would simply run like clockwork because there were excellent texts that said it was a good thing to do, there had been tentative backing from the UKCC (1996), and Trusts had a policy stating it was 'good practice'.

What is required, if the full benefits of supervision are going to be felt by supervised nurses and service users, is a sense that this process is a core activity which is not set aside or set up to be an ad-hoc luxury. In brief, it is a cultural shift, and the creation of a climate, not merely a task to be performed to satisfy an audit process.

It seems to me that there is some movement in this direction. Nursing is taking some steps to go beyond rhetorical aspirations and is striving to ensure that reflective practice and development can flourish, not just in academic settings where the phones don't ring and service users stay safely in case-studies. But in the midst of the clinical arena where the action takes place. A good example of this progress can be seen in the development of the Consultant Nurse role.

The Consultant Nurse and clinical supervision

There are detailed accounts elsewhere in this book regarding the development of the Consultant Nurse role. A key point that is, I believe, worth considering is that these roles are not simply an additional career choice for nurses but an acknowledgement that a cultural shift is a key factor if our aspirations are really about making a significant impact of clinical practice.

Manley (2000) highlights the importance of influencing the ethos of the clinical arena. What does this really mean? One thing we mean when we consider the notion of culture is as a substance that nurtures growth. This requires a degree of permanence, continuity or consistence. In this context, a major aim for Consultants Nurse is to foster a climate in which enthusiasm, enquiry and reflection are cardinal values. Manley (2000) goes on to specify key tasks that are viewed as critical in terms of changing the ethos in the clinical arena.

Clarifying values

The first task is that of 'values clarification'. Attempting to identify core beliefs that drive practice, and examining these principles to develop a commonly held, detailed view of what a given team aspires to. If we take this notion and examine it in the context of clinical supervision, there is a good fit. Dexter and Wash (1990) process model of clinical supervision maps out the path from reflecting upon a current clinical situation and establishing a detailed picture of progress.

Mapping and gapping

The second task identified here is that of identifying gaps between espoused values and action – or 'mapping and gapping'. Organisations and the sub systems within them deal with countless demands and expectations – some explicit, some less so. It is easy to foresee how this kind of complex and often obscure situation inevitably leads to erratic links between principles and practice. At one time or another we all face a choice between conforming to group behaviours which may at times be at odds with one's own principles, after all, the need to feel like we belong is a fundamental one. Nurses at all levels of an organisation make choices on the basis of what is the least worst option, given the lack of resources that may often be at a clinicians disposal.

Once again, if we think of this process of challenging incongruent, aspects of a culture well delivered supervision is a tool that does the job. The Consultant Nurse role is a strategic one. It is structured to tackle these details at the heart of practice that are extremely difficult to access from an operational management position focussed, as it inevitably must, on the effective deployment of scarce resources and the increasingly complex pursuit of political and organisational goals.

An additional concluding point made in Manley's work (2000), is that this process of clarifying and developing values needs to be evident on all levels of the clinical arena: practice areas as well as strategic forums. My view is that a Consultant Nurse is in a position to not only stay connected to the clinical field through the 'expert practice' function, but also to be able to form influential bonds and alliances with nursing colleagues as a result of this process, struggling with the same constraints, engaging in the same search for solutions (that don't always exist). In addition to being part of the work with patients which may often have a 'day to day' quality but can, when considered from the patients experience, have an enormous impact for the good or otherwise.

More than catharsis

These links can be explored and developed in clinical supervision into a powerful medium for developing a culture of reflection, enthusiasm and learning. We could probably get by with Consultants Nurses developing supervision methods that are safe, supportive and have a cathartic quality to them. This would be – I believe – a missed opportunity to utilise the wealth of talent that exists in the nursing profession, both for the direct participants of clinical supervision and for the most important people: the service users and their families.

An important difference in the development of the Consultant Nurse role is that it has been a strategic development. By and large, prior to this role, clinical developments of this nature relied largely on individuals championing a cause or a local development that gained the respect and resources of stakeholders in that area. Whilst much good clinical work was done in this way, there was a notable absence of central strategic leadership driving this process. The implication for innovative clinicians often simultaneously dealing with clinical, managerial and strategic issues themselves was that such developments weren't valuable unless they had an immediate impact upon the political priority of that day.

The inception of the Consultant Nurse role sends out a different message. It recognises the scope and potential of the nursing profession and also that nurses have the talents to assume this leadership role. More importantly, the Making a Difference strategy (DoH 2001) add up to a recognition that the clinical arena is not somehow subordinate to its managerial or academic counterparts, but worthy of developing as a rich and varied arena for practice development. In other words, the contribution of nursing not only counts, but is crucial at all levels.

Conclusion

In closing, it is clear that clinical supervision is prized by participants but is at a formative and complex developmental stage. It is, as yet, unclear whether the process of supervision actually has a positive impact on outcomes for service users and their carers. Clearly, further enquiry is called for to tackle this key question. The challenge to Consultants Nurses is to use their clinical, leadership and facilitative skills to influence the practice environment and accelerate the development of nursing. If this can be accomplished, then the process will be fruitful for clinicians and patients alike.

References

Barker P (1992) Psychiatric nursing. In: Butterworth T. *Clinical Supervision and Mentorship in Nursing*. London: Chapman and Hall.

Butterworth T. and Faugier J (1992) *Clinical Supervision and Mentorship in Nursing*. London: Chapman and Hall.

Butterworth T (1996) Clinical supervision – a hornet's nest ... or honey pot? *Nursing Times* 93(44), pp. 27–29.

Castledine G. (1994) What is clinical supervision? *British Journal of Nursing* 3(21), p. 1133.

Cutcliffe J and Proctor B (1998) An alternative training approach to clinical supervision. *British Journal of Nursing* 7(5), pp. 280–285.

Department of Health (2001) Making a difference the nursing, midwifery and health visiting contribution the midwifery action plan. London: HMSO.

Dexter G and Wash M (1995) *Psychiatric Nursing Skills: A Patient Centred Approach* (2nd edn) London: Chapman Hall.

Egan G. (1993) *The Skilled Helper*. 5th edn. California: Brookes/Cole.

Fisher M. (1996) Using reflective practice in clinical supervision. *Professional Nurse* 11(7), pp. 443–444.

Fowler J. (1995) Nurse's perception of the elements of good supervision. *Nursing Times* 91(22), 33–37.

Fowler J. (1996) How to use models of clinical supervision in practice. *Nursing Standard* 10(29), pp. 42–47.

Fowler J (1996) The organization of clinical supervision within the nursing profession: a review of the literature. *Journal of Advanced Nursing*, 23, pp. 471–478.

Goorapah D (1997) Clinical supervision. *Journal of Clinical Nursing*, 6, pp. 173–178.

Hawkins, P and Shohet R. (1994) *Supervision in the Helping Professions*. Milton Keynes: Open University.

Heron J. (1993) *Helping the Client*. London: Sage.

Hyrkas K., Koivula M. and Paunonen M. (1999) Clinical supervision in nursing in the 1990s – current state of concepts, theory and research. *Journal of Nursing Management*, 7, 177–187.

Johns C. (1993) Professional supervision. *Journal of Nursing Management*, 1 pp. 9–18.

Jones A (1997) A 'bonding between strangers': a Palliative Model of Clinical Supervision. *Journal of Advanced Nursing*, 26, pp. 1026–1035.

Manley K (2000) Organisational Culture and Consultant Nurse Outcomes: Part 1 Organisational Culture. *Nursing Standard* 24 May, 14(36), pp. 34–38.

Mezirow J (1981) Education for perspective transformation: women's re-entry programs in community colleges. In: Snowball J, Ross K and Murphy K (1994) Illuminating Dissertation Supervision Through Reflection. *Journal of Advanced Nursing*, 19, pp. 1234–1240.

Proctor B (1986) Supervision: a Co-operative Exercise in Accountability. In: Cutcliffe J and Proctor B (1998) An Alternative Training Approach to Clinical Supervision. *British Journal of Nursing*, 7(5), pp. 280–285.

Rogers C. (1967) *On Becoming A Person*. London: Constable.

Schon D (1987) Educating the reflective practitioner how professionals think in action. In: Andrews M (1996) Using Reflection to Develop Clinical Expertise. *British Journal of Nursing*, 5, pp. 508–513.

Snowball J, Ross K and Murphy K (1994) Illuminating dissertation supervision through reflection. *Journal of Advanced Nursing*, 19, pp. 1234–1240.

Wolsey P and Leach L (1997) Clinical supervision – a hornet's nest? *Nursing Times* 93(44), pp. 24–27.

CHAPTER TWELVE

Consultant Nurse: mental health nursing the mental health nurse?

Mick Norman

Introduction

I commenced my training to become a mental health, or psychiatric, nurse as it was termed in the vernacular of the day, in 1986. A decade or so later I found myself wandering around the career hinterland of mental health nursing, occupying a variety of positions around the level of 'G' grade, having witnessed the flight of colleagues into the heady world of academia, assorted quasi-nursing jobs outside the mainstream NHS, or disappearing into the realms of management. At the same time I encountered a reaction to this from colleagues who had remained at what they perceived to be the 'sharp end' of nursing, that is to say nursing of persons within hospital based environments. These nurses would frequently grumble during their 'hand-overs' about how community based nurses, academics, nurse managers, and the like, had lost touch with the reality of mental health nursing. Attempts at engagement by these 'senior nurses' were deemed to be evidence of a desire to justify apparent 'cushy' jobs involving lease cars, regular hours and access to academic courses which where perceived to be of little relevance to the day to day quest to find meaning to the problems-of-living that the persons-in-care entrusted to 'junior' colleagues by their medical colleagues presented with.

Over the ensuing 5 years I completed my CPN diploma, gained my first degree, moved Trusts and encountered my first real, live, Consultant Nurse. I had been aware of the Consultant Nurse, as a concept, for some time since the publication of the publication 'Guidelines on the role of the Consultant Nurse' (Department of Health, 1999). My first impressions back then had been that this new post had been designed for persons with no life outside nursing, being apparently expected to fulfil roles of research, teaching, clinical practice, advising nursing and non-nursing colleagues in addition presumably to undertaking their own activities of daily living!

This first exposure to a live Consultant Nurse coincided with my acceptance of my first true 'management' post within nursing. I was entrusted with the daily management of a Community Mental Health Team at a time of significant change. This state of flux revolved around the integration of health and social care services, with attendant cultural changes, as well as a plethora of Department of Health missives indicating at some length proposed functions and roles for teams such as ours. In addition to which the service locally was embarking upon the quest to operate within a 'whole-system', rather than the traditional watered-down medical model that had effectively stemmed from an apparent desire to replicate the psychiatric ward hierarchy, albeit within a building often situated in 'the community'.

The history of mental health nursing is arguably one of continued self-doubt and crisis of professional identity. This was undoubtedly a state I could identify with as I became involved in the day to day running of an 'integrated mental health care service'. In recent years this has been characterised by the debate over whom we should be seeking to help. On the one hand there has been the directives to focus our energies on those persons suffering from 'severe and enduring mental illness'. At the same time we have witnessed an increasing demand for attention from our medical colleagues in general practice to 'deal with' persons with problems of living such as generalised anxiety and low mood.

Within the ranks of mental health nursing itself we appear to have polarised camps. On the one hand the 'psycho-technologists' with their call for evidence based, psychosocial interventions, cognitive behavioural therapies, dialectical behavioural therapies, *et al.* At the other end of the continuum we have the more 'humanistic' school of mental health nursing, based around the concept of 'being with' rather than 'doing to' the person in care suffering from mental distress.

The introduction of the Consultant Nurse would appear to have highlighted this dichotomy further, in that on the one hand it has been seen as an 'expert' role, whose function is to enhance the technical skills of the mental health nurse further, with increased focus on the development of nursing skills in the aforementioned psycho-technologies. The alternative approach could be described as that of attempting to highlight and add clarity to the on-going debate over the role of the mental health nurse, through increasing the professional self-confidence of mental health nursing as a discreet discipline within the panoply of professions occupying the mental health field.

What are the skills of mental health nursing?

When attempting to define the skills of mental health nursing it is tempting to produce a list of techniques and tools, or what Barker (1999) calls 'psycho technologies', employed by the practising Registered Mental Nurse. Yet it occurred to me, as such a list began to evolve, that to categorise these as the 'skills' of mental health nursing is not dissimilar to defining a skilled joiner by describing the tools they use and what they are used for. Such a list would give no distinction between the highly skilled joiner and a keen 'do-it-yourself' enthusiast. A distinction between the professional joiner and enthusiastic amateur may be found in the level of knowledge about the material they use, the confidence they hold in using these tools and their ability to combine these to produce a functional, well-finished item, which is both durable and aesthetically pleasing.

This is not to imply that the identification of the tools and techniques used is not relevant to the question, but rather that an important element in the identification of the skills of mental health nursing is the recognition that the essence of skill lies primarily in the appropriate and timely use of these interventions. As Barker (2002) tells us, the essence of mental health nursing is not merely to 'address the immediate distress and disorder associated with psychiatric crisis'.

It may also be worth re-emphasising at this point that the aim of this section is the exploration of mental health nursing as a concept, rather than focusing on the work of mental health nurses. Much debate exists around the question of what group of persons-in-care mental health nursing should be working with (White, 1993, The Patients Association, 1994, Gourney and Brooking, 1995). This debate if primarily about whether mental health nursing should focus more on the group of persons-in-care suffering from primarily psychotic illnesses, with an emphasis on medication compliance, therapeutic interventions with the families of persons-in-care and specific psycho-social interventions (Gourney and

Sandford, 1998). I feel that although elements of this may be valuable to demonstrate some aspects of the use of the skills possessed by mental health nurses, it is not directly relevant to this discussion.

What is the focus of mental health nursing?

If mental health nursing skills are to be utilised effectively with any group of persons-in-care, then it may be worth attempting to define the focus of mental health nursing. The contents of the following discussion are primarily focused on the use of mental health nursing skills in the care of persons with physical illness, since this is a clinical area I have an interest in and was working in at the time the contents of the paper were conceived.

Barker (1999) suggests that as mental health nurses 'we have no real interest in people's disease or their health for that matter: instead, nurses are interested in people's relationship with their illness, or with their health'. He further suggests that mental health nursing is 'concerned with the challenge of promoting health when a person presents with some illness, disease, or dysfunction'.

These statements would appear to suggest that mental health nursing is not in itself about mental illness, but rather about enabling the person-in-care to deal with the consequences of their illness, disease or distress. If mental health nursing is 'the means by which nurses can help people to grow or move forward in their lives' (Barker and Jackson, 1997), then it would seem this may equally well be applied in the care of persons with physical illness.

Mental health nursing, as a separate branch of the profession of nursing, would appear to differ from other branches of nursing found in primary care by its special emphasis on the person-in-care's psychological, social and spiritual domain (Cutcliffe *et al.*, 2001). Mental health nursing as a concept is therefore concerned with using the skills of the nurse to promote these aspects of the person-in-care's well being through the utilisation of both existing and additional skills and techniques. The fundamental distinguishing feature is that where mental health nursing is focused on 'being with', the physical care based nursing domain is predominantly about 'doing to' (Cutcliffe *et al.*, 2001).

In some ways though, the focus of mental health nursing is apparently little different to that of other branches of nursing in that it has as its focus the human being, or person-in-care. However, Barker *et al.* (1997) cite Peplau as suggesting the subject of focus for mental health nursing includes 'a considerable array of dysfunctional human responses to gravely distressing human conditions'. These include 'anxiety, loneliness, changes in self-concept and grief as examples of human response patterns that nurses might observe, and respond to, during relationships with patients.'

The essence of mental health nursing's focus would appear to be an emphasis on the person-in-care's adaptation to their illness and the development of their abilities to utilise available opportunities to overcome perceived needs or deficits. From a pragmatic viewpoint, and for the purpose of this chapter, such a definition needs to be translated into a comprehensive framework that will indicate the qualities that mental health nursing as a concept possesses and which may be transferred into the care of persons with physical illness.

The qualities of mental health nursing

Mental health nursing is about 'caring *with* rather than caring *for* people, irrespective of the context of care' (Barker *et al.*, 1997). Mental health nursing has been described as 'an interactive, developmental human activity, more concerned with the future development of the person than with the origins or causes of their present mental distress' (Barker *et al.*, 1997).

As such it has been argued that mental health nursing, as a craft, has much in common with a number of other professional groupings within the field of counselling and psychotherapies (Wilshaw, 1997), in addition to those in other branches of nursing. Wilshaw (1997) identified this commonality as involving a number of issues. These include what he defined as 'curative factors' and 'core features of the helping relationship'. The essence of these appears to be encapsulating much of the quality of mental health nursing as discussed by a number of authors (Barker, 1997; Bowers and Crossling, 1994). They argue that essential to any therapeutic intervention is the relationship between the nurse and the person-in-care, with subsequent interventions being determined by this therapeutic relationship, whilst the particular clinical intervention employed also share a degree of commonality.

The helping, or therapeutic relationship, which arguably forms the core of mental health nursing, has been explored and defined by a number of authors from a variety of professional origins (Heron, 1990; Clarkson, 1994; Price, 1994). This relationship has been defined in a number of ways. Clarkson (1994) identified five modes of therapeutic relationship used in psychotherapy:

1. The working alliance.
2. The transferential/counter-transferential relationship.
3. The developmentally needed relationship.
4. The I–thou, or person-to-person relationship.
5. The transpersonal relationship.

Of these the most widely applied in mental health nursing is the 'working alliance', which takes the form of an understanding by both the helper and person-in-care of the work to be done, with a recognition of working to a common end. The working alliance model has been identified as possessing three elements: 'goals, bonds, and tasks' (Bordin, E. cited by Clarkson, P., 1994). When applied to mental health nursing the working alliance framework has been described as a 'bond of trust between nurse and client for the practice of high quality nursing'. (Haller, L. cited by Price, V., 1994).

The therapeutic bond has been identified as comprising of three components:

1. 'Role investment', or the degree of commitment by both parties.
2. Empathic resonance, or the way that the participants are in tune with one another.
3. Mutual affirmation, or the level of care and concern that each party has for the other.'

(Orlinsky *et al.* cited by Price, V. 1994)

Therapeutic goals originate from both those set by the nurse during the contact with the person-in-care, and those resulting from negotiating with the person-in-care, with a focus on what the desired achievement or outcome. Price (1994) suggests that 'the establishment of mutually agreed outcome goals between the client and mental health nurse can be seen to be fundamentally an activity which considers one of its primary functions to be the empowerment of others'.

Closely linked to the therapeutic goals are the therapeutic tasks. Once again, Price (1994) describes how 'it becomes the task of the mental health nurse, in their capacity as resource person, to map out to the client the rules of engagement governing the counselling process'. In addition to the explanatory role, this is seen to have an ethical dimension in that issues of confidentiality (Barker, 1997) and potential misuse or misinterpretation of the nurse's role within the relationship are covered (Moorey, 1998).

The second area of commonality described by Wilshaw (1997) which may be seen to be shared between mental health nursing and other inter-personal therapy providing professional groups is that of the 'curative fac-tor' found within the therapeutic process. These are effectively elements of the therapeutic process that may be identified as potential agents of therapeutic change. They have been identified as:

1. 'A basic matrix of good patient – therapist relationship resting on both real and fantasised qualities that each bring to their work together;
2. The release of emotional tension;
3. Cognitive learning or the acquisition of insight;
4. Operant conditioning by means of subtle and often non-verbal cues of approval and disapproval, as well as by corrective emotional experi-ences in the relationship;
5. Suggestion and persuasion, usually implicit, occasionally explicit;
6. Unconscious identification with the analyst, both conceptually and behaviourally: and
7. Repeated reality testing and 'working through'.'

(Marmor, 1982, cited in Wilshaw, G. 1997).

Wilshaw (1997) observes that this list does not indicate a preference for any particular therapeutic approach, but rather it refers to a process of engagement. He suggests that it may be argued that the process described may even go outside the domain of professional 'helping' to include ordi-nary helpful encounters between human beings' (Wilshaw, 1997).

The suggestion that mental health nursing is on a par with 'ordinary helpful encounters between human beings' is objectively descriptive of mental health nursing. Barker (1999) goes so far as to suggest that caring for people is actually about 'giving power back to the people or helping them to realise their own power in diverse ways'. It is arguable that the quality of mental health nursing lies in the use to which the nurse puts their *self*.

In identifying this concept of self, Wosket (1999) emphasises the important distinction between 'the *person* of the therapist and the therapist's *use of self*. The character of the therapist, whilst not inconsequential with the person-in-care, differs from the use of self in that the latter is an intentional therapeutic act with intended outcomes.

An interesting theory which goes some way to defining further both the quality of mental health nursing and why it differs subtly from ordinary human interaction is given by Heron (1990) when he suggests that: 'What makes the effective helper is an interaction between inner grace, character and cultural influence'. Heron defines grace as consisting of five attributes:

1. 'Warm concern for and acceptance of the other;
2. Openness and attunement to the other's experiential reality;
3. A grasp of what the other needs in the right manner for his or her essential flourishing;
4. An ability to facilitate the realisation of such needs in the right manner and at the right time; and
5. An authentic presence.'

(Heron, 1990)

Heron describes grace as being present in all humans, independent of professional training, which in turn may have either a positive or negative influence upon it. Grace manifests itself 'in terms of the norms, values and belief systems of the prevailing culture.' (Heron, (1990). Character is defined as what the person makes of himself or herself through interaction with this culture.

Applied to the concept of mental health nursing Heron's theory would seem to imply that although the training given, including formal educational techniques, has an influence on a person's grace, this is not in itself what produces an effective helper. It is the influence of peers and others in the socialisation into the role of the mental health nurse that enables the person's grace to flourish and in turn to be expressed individually through character. In terms of importance of these components it has been argued that the 'personal qualities (philosophy) of the therapist are significantly more important in enabling the growth of the client than the specific psychotherapeutic interventions'. (Rogers C. cited by Oxley P, 1996).

It would therefore seem that an argument exists to say that the essence of mental health nursing lies not in its psycho-technological repertoire, or status in the health care hierarchy, but is a culturally, individually and philosophically defined approach which aims to 'facilitate the individual's own problem-solving process in addressing their human dilemmas' (Oxley, 1996).

Personal reflections

So what has this to do with the title of this chapter – 'mental health nursing the mental health nurse'? Well, I would argue that if mental health nursing is primarily a process of facilitation, then this would appear to have much in common with definitions of the role of the Consultant Nurse.

Further discussion with both Consultant Nurse colleagues and other Mental Health Nurses has led me to identify a number of significant commonalities between both the relationships of nurse and the person-in-care, and the Consultant Nurse and Mental Health Nurse colleagues. I would acknowledge at this stage that this has been a primarily an anecdotal discourse, relying as it has on informal discussion and reflection with little recourse to any evidence base. None the less, in keeping with the theme of this chapter, I feel that such reflections promote thought and debate, rather than offer any definitive response to questions.

At this point, and in the spirit of the preceding sections of this chapter I would like to share with the reader a vision. This vision is of a mental health service in which the giving of care actually enhances the well being, both physically and psychologically, of the *caregiver*. Historically much has been written of the cost to the individual caregiver in terms of resultant negative states of work related stress and 'burn-out' (Payne and

Firth-Cozens, 1987, cited by Carson, *et al.*, 1995). In this envisaged 'brave new world' the mental health nurse finds and develops aspects of themselves, both professional and personal, through the process of 'being with' the person-in-care through their journey to improved mental well-being. Community based mental health nurses will eagerly await fresh referrals and allocations meetings, whilst ward based staff will long for the telephone call announcing an impending admission.

> 'You may say I'm a dreamer,
> but I'm not the only one'

John Lennon (1971)

The cynics amongst you, of which mental health nursing has more than its fair share, may be declaring statements similar to those in Mr. Lennon's lyrics. However, as the man points out on a later track of the same album, no matter how well 'you may shine your shoes and wear a suit…. one thing you can't hide, is when you're crippled inside' (Lennon, J. 1971). So how do we reach the nirvana of a service, which is a joy to work in, and a source of bountiful personal growth? Whilst not wishing to put my Consultant Nurse colleagues in a position where they are besieged by hordes of stressed Mental Health Nurses eager to learn the secret of eternal professional self-fulfilment, I will at this stage be so bold as to suggest that part of the answer could, and I stress the word *could*, be through the role of the Consultant Nurse in mental health.

How so?

At this point I shall revert to my original premise of the Consultant Nurse being the mental health nurse's mental health nurse. The first stage will be for the Consultant Nurse to have the courage to descend from any ivory tower they have located for use as their comfort zone and begin to communicate with their mental health-nursing colleagues. This may be described as building a therapeutic relationship with their 'person-in-care', whether through attending team/ward meetings or through work-ing clinically alongside nursing colleagues. They will need to find out about the hopes and fears of their colleagues, what their world-view is, how they perceive their situation to be, while all the time having the patience not to wade in offering suggestions or advice. 'Being with', rather than 'doing to' (Cutcliffe *et al.*, 2001).

As in the process of nursing a distressed person-in-care, this initially may feel extremely uncomfortable for the Consultant Nurse, since, as in mental health nursing, the temptation is there to try to solve the person-in-care's problems for them, with little regard to the effect this may have on their future coping strategies. However, as Barker (1997) emphasises, the initial assessment role is to try 'to gain an overall picture, one that describes positive characteristics as well as problems'. Obviously, should there be any outstanding issues which are felt to be a danger to the mental health nurse professionally or personally, these should be dealt with urgently, but even then care should be taken to avoid any risk of dis-empowering the mental health nurse with consequent adverse effects on their professional self-esteem.

Once an understanding of the issues understood, these should be fed back to the mental health nurse, avoiding any possible mis-interpretation of being a patronising, interfering, know-it-all. Use of cognitive re-framing techniques will come in useful here. Should this be achieved then the working alliance (Haller, L. cited by Price, V., 1994) may begin to be achieved. Through this 'working alliance' a 'therapeutic bond' with the mental health nurse may be made with the Consultant Nurse, in much the same way as described by Orlinsky *et al.* (cited by Price, V., 1994).

At this stage it may be worth reminding Consultant Nurses that they potentially hold a position of power previously unknown to nurses. Many will have key roles in the NHS Trusts and organisations they work in. They hold positions which have the potential to influence the policy makers within the Trusts which employ their mental health nursing colleagues, and often have direct communication with trust directors and senior managers. As such they hold a responsibility to be advocates for their mental health-nursing colleagues. It may be that this level of power feels strange and unusual for those with a nursing background. To fight shy of this though, effectively does a dis-service to nursing.

Clinical supervision is a vitally important process which keeps the person-in-care safe. Clinical supervision by peers, and others in senior nursing positions, is of the utmost importance should the Consultant Nurse wish to establish and maintain a credible and important role in mental health nursing.

'And then one day you find,
10 years have got behind you'

Pink Floyd (1973)

So where does this leave the future of the Consultant Nurse in Mental Health? Before too long the role of the Consultant Nurse will no longer be a novelty and will be an integral part of nursing's professional career structure. If the role is to become a valued one for nurses, and not just a historical dinosaur, then the role of being the Mental Health Nurse's Mental Health Nurse will need to evolve and develop. For this evolution to be of use to Mental Health Nurses it is important that acknowledgement is made of the influence of external, societal, factors in this process, just as the role of the Mental Health Nurse has changed through the influence of factors outside the immediate cosy world of Psychiatry. I envisage such changes as being gradual, though already we as a profession have embraced the move to community-based care, integration with our social care colleagues, and potentially the development of roles previously the preserve of medicine – such as prescribing. With awareness of this process Mental Health Nursing may harness their influence for the benefit of both the profession and their persons-in-care. Mental health Nursing has a proud record of embracing change and responding positively to the challenges presented to it.

Identification of these changes may occur through on-going dialogue between Consultant Nurses and Mental Health Nursing colleagues. Through their access to the higher levels of health service management and governmental departments, Consultant Nurses are potentially well placed to foresee these changes and therefore significantly impact on nursing. In much the same manner as the Mental Health Nurse is able to develop an on-going helping relationship with the person-in-care suffering from an enduring mental illness, the skilled Consultant Nurse will be able to utilise this relationship to promote professional growth, both individually and to nursing as a whole.

Conclusion

As a practising Community Mental Health Nurse and Nurse Manager, I hold the hope that much of the preceding discussion strikes appropriate chords and holds no fears for my Consultant Nurse colleagues. For those Consultant Nurses who hold doubts I would hymn:

> 'Turn around, go back down,
> back the way you came'

> Quicksilver Messenger Service (1967)

If the role of the Consultant Nurse is to achieve lasting credibility within the ranks of Mental Health Nursing then the temptation to distance itself from the 'grass roots' of the profession must be avoided at all costs. In the same way as the Mental Health Nurse needs to recognise the common humanity which bonds them to the person-in-care, so must the Consultant Nurse recognise and embrace both the common background and hopes for the future which they hold with their nursing colleagues. If Consultant Nurses take the avenue of professional superiority then as surely as persons-in-care disengage with unhelpful services, then so will Mental Health Nurses perceive Consultant Nurses to be an historical irrelevancy, with similar dis-engagement. Should such a situation occur, I see little hope for any assertive outreach to aid professional re-engagement!

References

Barker, P. (1999) *The Philosophy and Practice of Psychiatric Nursing.* London. Churchill Livingstone.

Barker, P. (2002) Realising the promise of liaison mental health care. In Regal, S. and Roberts, D. (eds.) *Mental Health Liaison – a handbook for nurses and health professionals.* Edinburgh. Bailliere Tindall. pp. 3–21.

Barker, P. and Jackson, S. (1997) mental Health Nursing: making it a primary concern. *Nursing Standard.* 11. (17) 15 January, pp. 39–41.

Bowers, L. and Crossling, P. (1994) Skills training in community psychiatric nurse education. *Mental Health Nursing.* April, 14(2).

Carson, J. Bartlett, H. Fagin, L. Brown, D. and Leary, J. (1995) Stress and the community psychiatric nurse. In: Brooker, C. and White, E. (eds) *Community psychiatric nursing: a research perspective–Volume 3.* London: Chapman & Hall.

Clarkson, P. (1994) The psychotherapeutic relationship. In: Clarkson, P. and Pokorny, M. (eds.) *The handbook of psychotherapy.* London: Routledge, pp. 28–48.

Cutcliffe, J. Black, C. Hanson, E. and Goward, P. (2001) The commonality and synchronicity of mental health nurses and palliative care nurses: closer than you think? Part one. *Journal of Psychiatric and Mental Health Nursing.* 8, pp. 53–59.

Department of Health (1999) *Guidelines on the role of the Consultant Nurse.* London: HMSO.

Gournay, K. and Brooking, J. (1995) The community psychiatric nurse in primary care: an economic analysis. In: Brooker, C. and White, E. (eds) *Community Psychiatric Nursing: a research perspective–volume 3.* London: Chapman and Hall.

Gournay, K. and Sandford, T. (1998) Training for the workforce. In: Brooker, C. and Repper, J. (eds) *Serious Mental Health Problems in the Community: Policy, Practice and Research.* London: Bailliere Tindall.

Heron, J. (1990) *Helping the Client: a creative practical guide.* London: Sage.

Lennon, J. (1971) Plastic Ono Band (with the flux fiddlers). *Imagine.* Apple Records, UK.

Moorey, J. (1998) The ethics of professional care. In: Barker, P. and Davidson, B. (eds) *Psychiatric Nursing: ethical strife.* London: Arnold.

Oxley, P. (1996) The skilled practitioner: nature or nurture? *Mental Health Nursing,* 16(1), January, pp. 6–7.

Patients Association (1994) Mental health nursing: a spectrum of skills. *Mental Health Nursing,* 14(3), June, pp. 6–8.

Pink Floyd (1973) *Time.* EMI, UK.

Price, V. (1994) Building a therapeutic alliance when counselling clients. *Mental Health Nursing,* 14(6), December.

Quicksilver Messenger Service (1967) *Pride of Man.* Capitol Records: USA.

White, E. (1993) Community psychiatric nursing 1980 to 1990: a review of organisation, education and practice. In: Brooker, C. and White, E. (eds) *Community psychiatric nursing: a research perspective–volume 2.* London: Chapman and Hall.

Wilshaw, G. (1997) Integration of therapeutic approaches: a new direction for mental health nurses? *Journal of Advanced Nursing,* 26, pp. 15–19.

Wosket, V. (1999) *The therapeutic Use of Self: counselling practice, research and supervision.* London: Routledge.

CHAPTER THIRTEEN

Integration of therapeutic approaches

Keeping sight of what really helps in mental health care

Gary Wilshaw

Introduction

In this chapter, I will discuss the value of the Consultant Nurse taking up the stance of a specific therapeutic school as a basis for practice in mental health nursing, such as cognitive behavioural therapy or patient centred therapy. This is viewed against a background of increased interest in 'non-purist' forms of therapeutic approach in the fields of psychotherapy and counselling.

The common factors present in effective helping relationships are highlighted along with a way of understanding the fundamental *form* of a given helping relationship which is perhaps independent of theoretical orientation (Clarkson, 1992). Thinking in this mode may cut across traditional 'models of nursing/therapy' thinking, and may assist the Consultant Nurse in addressing the core issues when considering sustainable practice development. This thinking may allow mental health nurses in general to adopt appropriate patient need driven interventions, which are not hamstrung by theoretical dogma. Given this, I will suggest an 'honourable position' of theoretical eclecticism for the Consultant Nurse in mental health, for nurse education and practice in general.

Background

Integration of therapeutic approaches and theory has become an increasingly important and widespread concept in the literature in recent years

An earlier version of this chapter was published as Wilshaw, G. (1997) Integration of therapeutic approaches: a new direction for mental health nurses? *Journal of Advanced Nursing*, 26, pp. 15–19.

(Mahrer, 1989), influencing the thinking of many workers in varied fields of nursing, counselling, psychotherapy and clinical psychology. 'Newer' therapeutic approaches such as Cognitive Analytic Therapy (CAT) (Ryle & Kerr, 2002) claim to be integrative, blending – in this case – core theory from both cognitive and psychodynamic schools. CAT is proving to be popular and attractive to nurses and other mental health care workers, perhaps because of its utility and reflection of the essentially pragmatic nature of many such staff groups and the work environment they operate within.

Norcross & Arkowitz (in Dryden & Grencavage, 1992) identify a 'common goal' in post-modern developments in therapy, that is to integrate therapies or at least to develop a coherent eclecticism. Attempts to integrate have been reported under the terms of eclecticism, integration, pluralism, rapprochement, unification and prescriptionism. In this chapter, I will set out to examine how some of these issues may offer a meaningful framework for the systematic and deliberate use of the helping relationship to mental health nurses.

The above authors cite an increasing dissatisfaction with so called 'pure' forms of therapeutic approach, and hint at a limitation on thinking and practice that may be brought to bear by remaining within the confines of a given therapeutic discipline. Norcross & Grencavage (1990), referring to this dissatisfaction, argue that there may increasingly be an acceptance of the possibility that no one approach is 'clinically adequate for all the problems, patients and situations' which the professional may come across. The authors go on to suggest that the enormous complexities encountered when looking at psychologically oriented difficulties demand such a range of possible responses and interventions that a singular approach is unlikely to suffice. Oddly, nursing may have both benefited and suffered from this apparent theoretical and practical disintegration. On the benefiting side, many nurses have been active in recent years in searching out training in what seemed/claimed to be 'useful' therapy approaches, thus adding new instruments to their eclectic toolkit. This may place nurses in a position of special receptivity and openness to integrationist thinking. On the negative side, there may have been a price to pay for the pursuit of multiple, perhaps incongruous trainings, not all of which may be learned in depth, and not all of which may make for a theoretically coherent basis for practice.

The healthy struggle to establish a therapeutic stance on professional practice continues today in mental health nursing even after more than two decades of exposure to 'nursing models', which have failed to maintain a visibility or presence in the minds of many practising nurses. In many ways this matter has a new urgency for the Consultant Nurse, given the claims of evidence of efficacy of specific intervention style with a specific patient need or problem. A clear example of this might be the relevance of cognitive behavioural interventions with the severely mentally ill (Bentall, 1996). An issue here is that 'nursing' requires the mental health nurse to be *more* than a cognitive behavioural therapist, and the therapeutic approach might be the one of choice at a given point in a very complex portfolio of activity, perhaps with a varied caseload with patients offering a range of challenges to the services.

The era of the 'guru' in the psychotherapies, when charismatic (usually) men led a school of thought that became a doctrine, is rightly viewed with increasing scepticism (Norcross & Grencavage, 1990). Each of the best known schools have attracted severe and fundamental criticism at some time, which perhaps at best weaken their position as a theoretical stance. The easiest examples of this to point to might be the lack of empirical substance to the theoretical backbone of psychodynamics; and in the cognitive behavioural arena – the fundamental assumption that (e.g. by Ellis, 1977) that cognitive content and process will take precedence and dictate Affect (Norcross & Grencavage, 1990).

Is one therapeutic approach 'better' than another?

In recent decades, writers have begun to suggest that the beneficial effects noted when patients receive care in a therapeutic relationship may be due in part to *common elements* that run across therapies – I shall say more about this later in this chapter. What this line of research suggests is that the evidence for significant differentials of therapeutic effect across different therapies is not always as strong as may be claimed. Bergin & Lambert *et al.* (1978) examined outcome indicators over a range of therapeutic styles and approaches reveal little differences and few reasons to suspect the greater efficacy of one approach over another. Miller *et al.* (1997) concluded that crucial variables such as *collaboration* are the elements that make a difference, rather than the 'badged' approach itself.

Byrne (1994) looked at the help being given to people with Schizophrenia, and found, as Miller & Powers (1988) had before her, that the instillation of a sense of *hope* was critical to positive coping. Again this is not the province of a particular approach, but may be a by-product of a composure and confidence that is conferred when a worker has a framework that they have belief in. In a similar vein, Cooper & Murray (2000) failed to support the efficacy of one specific psychological approach (including cognitive behavioural therapy) over another in the care and treatment of post-natal depression. In this case, as in others, researchers commonly report the centrality of non-specific *support*, given consistently over a sustained period of weeks (Holden *et al.*, 1989; Whitberg & Hwang, 1996).

Therapeutic 'tools' and applied helping processes – apparently from differing therapeutic schools – take place in the therapeutic relationship, and are sometimes known by different names, yet they overlap significantly. An example are the notions of transference in psychodynamic traditions, and that of unfinished business in Gestalt, game playing in Transactional Analysis and reciprocal roles in CAT. These concepts are distinct in that on the surface they have different origins and explanations, but in practice their use as tools of thinking and reflecting seem often to be interchangeable.

Out of the sort of awareness mentioned, the notion has developed that it may be appropriate to *address the commonalities* in developing therapeutic approaches, rather than to continue to add to the list of therapeutic options by the development of 'new' therapies. Indeed there is evidence that there is great interest in integration and commonalities within the broader community of professional helpers. Mahrer (1989) reports on studies indicating that up to a half of therapists in the nineteen seventies and eighties claimed to operate in some way reflective of an eclectic or integrative style. In my own work with mental health nurses in recent years, I have found that the vast majority are attempting to apply a range of therapeutic options on an 'as-needed' basis following assessment. It is rare – understandably – to find a mental health nurse defending a purist stance in a non-specialist post. Instead, experienced professionals often report the need to be able to 'move' between at least two theoretical and practical standpoints, often whilst identifying a 'homebase' set of key beliefs about the nature of personhood (for instance

– the belief that given the right environment and support, a person can usually find appropriate solutions to difficulties).

What are the 'curative factors' in the therapeutic process?

One approach to thinking about the features of the therapeutic encounter that are helpful, is offered by Marmor (1982). He suggests that seven elements exist which are the change-producing forces in therapy. They are:

1. A basic matrix of good patient-therapist relationship resting on both real and fantasised qualities that each bring to their work together.
2. The release of emotional tension.
3. Cognitive learning or the acquisition of insight.
4. Operant conditioning by means of subtle and often non-verbal cues of approval and disapproval, as well as by corrective emotional experiences in the relationship.
5. Suggestion and persuasion, usually implicit, occasionally explicit.
6. Unconscious identification with the analyst, both conceptually and behaviourally.
7. Repeated reality testing and 'working through' the issue/s.

It can be seen that the features listed do not 'belong' to any given theoretical stance. Instead, Marmor refers to processes that cut across disciplines and maybe even go outside the domain of professional 'helping' and include ordinary helpful encounters between human beings.

Perhaps picking up on these same sentiments in the broader context, Norcross & Grencavage (1990) point out the emergence of a systematic attempt to develop the notion of integration through the formation of interdisciplinary bodies devoted to that cause, an example being the Society for the Exploration of Psychotherapeutic Integration (SEPI). In addition, the proliferation of publications on the area, and interest reflected in seminar and conference agendas are cited as evidence of the growing importance in the movement.

Core features of the helping relationship

Clarkson & Lapworth (1992), in addressing the issue of commonalities in therapeutic schools, point to their recognition of *Physis*. First named by the ancient Greeks, it refers to a 'general creative force in evolution', and is paralleled by the authors with the general healing force in psychotherapeutic activity. Clarkson & Lapworth underline once more that this healing force seems to be located within the core of the helping relationship rather than the 'particular theory espoused'.

In the same paper, Clarkson and her colleague point to the importance of the background societal 'views of the person' in determining the theoretical constructs that might then develop in explaining and thinking about the experience of that person. These views are unconscious – or at least inexplicit – attitudes about what 'makes people tick', which are the unsurprising and organic products of contemporary thought and habits. Examples of this might be the evolution of behavioural perspectives during times of heavy and prolific industrial development – as in the middle of the 20th century, or the development of the cognitive or information processing models during the 'computer age'. Here, the predominant socially and commercially valued systems of thinking about man and the world understandably influence new constructs. This is an important point because it alerts us to the dangers of over-confidence in believing our own press on 'what works' in therapy, simply because our very understanding of what '*what works*' means, will be determined by the fickle and prevailing values of the time and culture.

In perhaps condensing the essence of the nature of the helping relationship, Clarkson (1994) purports five key 'types' of therapeutic relationship, and describes them as below. Clarkson's concepts are included here because they seem to offer a useful tool in the auditing of the subjective experience of current clinical relationships. In doing this, mental health nurses may be able to identify theoretical foundation stones of their central clinical tool – that is, their *relationship* with the patient.

1. *The working alliance*, which describes a contractually based 'agreement' or understanding between the parties on the work in hand, or a commitment to press ahead in some way with a spirit of working to some common end.

2. *The Transferential/Countertransferential relationship* describes a rich relationship when the central material worked with seems to be dynamic material that the patient (and nurse) brings, which then replicates/repeats itself within the nurse-patient relationship. Here, the nurse uses conscious awareness of the processes in an effort to develop insight and the ability to help by the informed choice of intervention.

3. The *developmentally needed relationship* is where the relationship has a corrective/reparative function, almost parental in nature, sometimes attempting to put right problems developed in dysfunctional developmental relationships earlier.

4. The *person-to-person relationship* is named, and compared to Buber's (1970) concept of 'I and thou'. Here, the predominant subjective experience of the helper is a person-to-person existential encounter. The helping relationship here is about the provision of a relationship and forum in which a partnership of exploration of this meeting can occur.

5. There is the *Transpersonal* relationship. This takes on board the spiritual element of the relationship and the sentiment that there may well be limits to what is 'knowable' about what any 'illness' is, what their relationship means and how it operates. Nurse and patient work toward an acceptance of this, and sense of shared wonder and openness to the experience and where it may lead.

Clarkson, 1994, pp. 28–48

Levels of integration

By this point, the reader may be asking questions of their own practice, and maybe the *degree* of any integration represented therein. To help, the work of Norcross & Arkowitz (1992) identifies three popular 'routes' to integration, which they say is detectable in the literature on the subject and in practice:

1. *Technical eclecticism*
   This describes a pragmatic approach in which the therapist or nurse seeks to select and use the approach that can demonstrably help the

patient. This is a evidence based judgement and takes account of what has worked before in an empirical sense, both for the particular person and in the broader literature.

2. *Theoretical integration*

This requires the integration of two or more theories of helping, with the aim that the resulting model will be better that the sum of the parts. This approach hints at more than a mere *blending* of complementary theories and practices. The goal is to create a synthesised and developed model that opens up new conceptualisations and avenues for thinking in practice and in research. A fairly recent example of a claimed theoretical integration is the development of CAT (Ryle & Kerr, 2002).

3. *Common factors*

This approach, as the title indicates, seeks to identify *commonalities* across approaches, in the belief that these commonalities may be instrumental in dictating outcome. This work is referred to earlier in this chapter in the context of comments by Marmor (1982), and others.

The practice of this Consultant Nurse

These perspectives will now be used to briefly reflect on the sort of approaches I would identify in my own clinical work. Like many of my mental healthcare colleagues, I have a sense of a 'home base' from which my practice grows and is conceptualised. This is likely to be related to training and supervision experiences over the years, and may even rest in more fundamental views about the human condition drawn from influences in my upbringing, reading and culture. My own particular 'home base' is rooted in the psychodynamic tradition but also contains powerful humanistic elements such as an acknowledgement about the effects of both over and under-socialisation (see Nelson Jones, 2001, below) and the development of effective coping styles. These beliefs reveal themselves in practice, record keeping, supervision and theoretical formulation of casework.

Having said this, I also have an awareness of the 'use' of particular interventions or approaches from other disciplines, *as a way of helping or responding* to a given situation. This suggests a *technical eclecticism* as outlined above, in that there is a certain pragmatism and 'right tools for the job' feel to many encounters with the patient. Here, clinical interventions are 'selected' within an 'evidence-based' framework, drawing upon knowledge of patient preferences, my preferences, and insights from research and publications where this is available. My work may be criticised as being no more than a 'patchwork' of therapeutic styles. However, to continue with the metaphor, when my practice feels to be at its best quality there is also a sense of 'seamlessness' in the use of these approaches. On many occasions, my subjective evidence is of an absorption of the approaches into the fabric of the relationship as a whole, and of my own individuality. This latter point has, over many years, led to my interest in the possibility of being truly authentic in therapeutic encounters.

In my experience there is an ease of integration of particular therapeutic approaches over others. This may relate to the 'commonality' issue discussed above and suggest a greater commonality or roots of origin between these approaches. Nelson-Jones (2001) for example, explores what he refers to as the 'stables' within which given approaches to helping emanate from. In looking at Humanistic approaches, a distinction is made between:

- *Humanistic – Perceptual*
  (Including person-centredness.) This stable emphasises the role of over-socialisation in the hindering of people's capacity to perceive themselves and their environment accurately. The key traditions of Rogerian therapy, Transactional Analysis and Gestalt are thought by the author to be within this category.

- *Humanistic – Rational*
  Also acknowledges the role of over-socialisation, but tends to concentrate on *under*-socialisation in the form of the lack of a development of 'how to' skills, helpful defences and thinking strategies. Rational Emotive Therapy (Ellis, 1977) Cognitive Behavioural Therapy (Beck, 1976) are the best known examples of approaches in this stable.

Given this, the use of awareness informed by knowledge of Trans-actional Analysis or Gestalt for example, within an essentially humanistic or Rogerian basis for helping seems plausible. Overall, it may be reasonable to expect the existence of a technical eclecticism that has a distinct pragmatism but is *not* just a 'tool selecting' exercise in some mechanical sense, which may ignore the context of the relationship as a whole.

Theoretical integration as described by Norcross & Arkowitz (1992) requires theoretical construction and synthesis in the sense of the creation of a *new* model for practice. CAT (Ryle & Kerr, 2002) is an example of a model that claims theoretical integration of psychodynamic and cognitive models.

Therapeutic schools – how similar are the differences?

The *Common Factors* movement is of interest in that the notion of a common thread or base within approaches to helping may well help explain my own, and perhaps that of the reader's subjective experience of being able to hold more than one tradition within what is felt to be a coherent relationship.

Within the psychodynamic approach, it is perhaps fair to say that a degree of 'expertise' is assumed by the professional in terms of attempting to know 'what is going on' in the relationship. This involves the formulation of 'theories' about the patient and attempts to 'explain' or interpret their position or difficulties. Patient-centredness on the other hand would place greater emphasis upon the patient being an 'expert on himself' (Nelson-Jones, 2001) the therapeutic 'work' being the facilitation of the climate by the helper in which the patients natural actualising or growth can take place, as opposed to the activity of expert-theorisation in a rather instrumental and removed sense.

However in spite of the differences, commonalities are not difficult to see. Both traditions have some common roots as mentioned above, (Nelson-Jones, 2001) value the individual, and require the development of a therapeutic alliance or partnership, and the working to an agreed if sometimes elusive goal. Both value the 'use of self' in that the helper attends to and makes active use of their internal subjective experience, albeit this occurring within the congruence of the humanistically oriented relationship as opposed to the opacity of the psychodynamic professional.

Conclusions

This discussion around therapeutic integration in nursing is offered as a contribution to debate about the therapeutic nature of mental health nursing and the basis of practice for nurses. There are implications for clinical practice, leadership, training at both pre and post-registration levels, and also for the structure of therapeutic opportunities in services. Effective services offer needs-based help that allows for the appropriate connection of those with skills, to those people who may benefit from those skills. This in turn requires that services be quite clear in their *therapeutic function*, and that the nurses (and others) who staff these services have the theoretical and practical basis to *deliver* the function.

There are one or two other obvious implications arising from this debate. Firstly, the 'commonalities' argument powerfully puts forward the notion that 'curative factors' within the helping traditions may be to do with *core elements*, rather that specific wisdom within any given approach. Given this, some transfer of learning to the work and development of the mental health nurse may be pertinent. Curative factors are seen by some to exist within and around the very process of the helping relationship. They describe and capture features of an energy which is deeply personal as opposed to technical, and evoke the essential nature of nursing as a caring art – concerned more with assisting people to cope and adjust than with 'cure' or the 'resolution of symptoms'.

Secondly, a version of a *technical eclecticism* could well be an honourable position for the Consultant Nurse mental health nurses to adopt in practice and thinking. The foundations for this may well be explained within the commonalities of approaches argument. If for a moment, the theoretical divisions between approaches are suspended in one's mind, and the possibilities of the importance of commonalities accepted, then the 'appropriate use' of interventions from various (coherent) styles are perhaps reduced to a much less worrying significance. Being drawn from different traditions, these interventions might become simply creative ways of 'being' in the given relationship that are responses to a fundamental desire to understand and help. It is my view that mental health nurses have long had a talent for the pragmatic and realistic use of approaches that may help the patient at a given point, and that this stance is both sensible and theoretically defensible.

References

Berne E (1964) *Games People Play* Penguin: London.

Bentall R P (1996) From cognitive studies of psychosis to cognitive behavioural therapy for psychotic symptoms, pp. 1–27. In: *Cognitive Behavioural Interventions With Psychotic Disorders*. Haddock G & Slade PD, Routledge: London.

Barker P (1985) Promoting growth through community mental health nursing. *Mental Health Nursing* May 1995, 15(3).

Barrowclough C & Tarrier N (1992) *Families of Schizophrenic Patients* Chapman & Hall: London.

Beck AT (1976) *Cognitive Therapy and the Emotional Disorders* New American Library: New York

Bergin AE & Lambert MJ (1978) The Evaluation of Therapeutic Outcomes. In: Garfield SL and Bergin AE (eds) *Handbook of Psychotherapy and Behaviour Change* Brunner/Mazel: New York.

Buber M (1970) *I and Thou* T & T Clark: Edinburgh.

Clarkson P (1994) The psychotherapeutic relationship. In: Clarkson P & Pokorny M (eds) *The Handbook of Psychotherapy* pp. 28–48. Routledge: London.

Clarkson P & Lapworth P (1992) Systemic integrative psychotherapy, pp. 41–83. In: Dryden W (1992) (ed.) *Integrative and Eclectic Therapy – a Handbook*. Open University Press: Bristol.

Cooper PJ, Murray L (2000) A controlled trial of the long-term effect of psychological treatment of post-partum depression: impact on maternal mood. *British Journal of Psychiatry* 183, pp. 77–84.

Dryden W (ed.) (1992) *Integrative and Eclectic Therapy – a Handbook*. Open University Press: Bristol.

Egan G (1985) *The Skilled Helper*. Brooks-Cole: California.

Ellis A (1977) The theory of rational emotive therapy. In: Ellis A & Grieger R (eds) *Rational Emotive Therapy,* Springer: New York.

Ellis A (1977) The basic clinical theory of rational emotive therapy. In: Ellis A & Grieger R (eds) *Handbook of Rational Emotive Therapy* Springer: New York.

Heron J (1990) *Helping the Patient*. Sage: London.

Holden JM, Sagovsky R, Cox JL (1989) Counselling in a general practice setting – controlled study of health visitor intervention in treatment of post-natal depression. *British Medical Journal* 298(6668) pp. 223–226.

Lloyd H (1993) Past, present, future – community psychiatric nursing and general practice. *Community Psychiatric Nursing Journal,* April, 13(2).

Mahrer A (1989) *The Integration of Psychotherapies, a Guide for Practising Therapists*. Human Sciences Press: New York.

Marmor J (1982) Change in psychoanalytic treatment, p. 66. In: Slipp (ed.) *Curative Factors in Dynamic Psychotherapy*. McGraw Hill: New York.

Miller SD, Duncan B L, Hubble MA (1997) *Escape from Babel: Towards a Unifying Language for Psychotherapy Practice*. Norton, New York.

Norcross JC & Arkowitz H (1992) The evolution and current status of psychotherapy integration pp. 1–40. In: Dryden W (ed.) (1992) *Integrative and Eclectic Therapy – a Handbook*. Open University Press: Bristol.

Norcross JC & Grencavage L (1990) Eclecticism and integration in counselling and psychotherapy: major themes and obstacles, pp. 1–33. In: Dryden W & Norcross JC (eds) *Eclecticism and Integration in Counselling and Psychotherapy*. Gale Publications: London.

Nelson Jones R (2001) 3rd edn. *The Theory and Practice of Counselling Psychology*. Cassell: London.

Rogers C (1965) *Patient Centred Therapy* Constable: London.

Ryle A, Kerr I (2002) *Introducing Cognitive Analytic Therapy*. Wiley, London.

Strupp H (1973) On the basic ingredients of psychotherapy. *Journal of Clinical And Consulting Psychology*, 41, pp. 1–8.

Whitberg B, Hwang CP (1996) Counselling of postnatal depression: a controlled study of a population based Swedish sample. *Journal of Affective Disorders*, 39(3) pp. 209–216.

CHAPTER FOURTEEN

What really helps in the process of recovery

Sallie Cooper

Introduction

I am a 'service user' of twelve years' experience including many acute in-patient admissions. I am also a 'people watcher', and the experiences and observations below are not all my own but have been absorbed and collated from other patients over the years. If you are a professional, you may feel that a glance at my headings, below, suggest to you that the material is too 'basic' and not for you. However, I would ask you to take a few minutes to consider my views as a product of insights gained over more than a decade.

When asked by the editor if I would like to contribute to this book, I readily agreed for two key reasons. The first is that I believe – as you might guess – that I have something to say that is worth the consideration of Consultant Nurses and others who may read this book. In sharing my views with this audience, I hope that they will be considered carefully and taken 'on board', perhaps treated as good quality 'data' alongside other forms of 'evidence' that I know modern healthcare systems to be hungry for! The second reason is that I have always tried to be open and constructive about both my 'health problems', and my experiences in having them responded to by healthcare systems. This chapter is thus a new development of this latter personal style, and one that I embrace with interest.

The ideas I want to put forward are intended to set out a range of key ideas that really make a difference to the quality of care a patient may experience. I have chosen to focus on those ideas that are *positive*, and capable of being embraced or considered by both professionals and *services* alike.

What really helps

Being treated as an intelligent equal

It is so easy to look at another person's problems and to see the way they should go, or what would 'help' them, then to break it down into small steps so they can understand and take the necessary action. I have had this done to me so many times and I find it insultingly patronising. I know there is no single answer, and that I will have to find answers for myself before I can own them. This is best done on equal terms with the professional concerned. (And don't ever forget that I, too, am a professional having had a lifetime's preparation – (training) – and many years' full-time experience.) I **know** how it feels to be a patient – something I hope you will never really know. I work from the premise that everyone is equal and that we all bring a fresh perspective to share. There is no room for 'us and them' in the world of recovery from mental illness.

Honesty, mutual respect and trust

These may seem obvious, but they are not easy for many patients who have a past they are used to hiding, and maybe fairly catastrophic experiences of sharing their lives verbally in the past.

If one starts with a premise of honesty and mutual respect things are more likely to evolve that way than if an air of suspicion reigns. I have experienced both, and I know when I am trusted I live up to that trust and if that trust is not expected it is much harder to establish boundaries for myself.

Trust can be expected first and then built upon, but if not expected, boundaries crumble. Far more is at stake for the patient if he/she is not trusted than for the professional.

Establishing firm boundaries at the outset is really important. Trust has to be earned. Experiences of fragility make one cautious of opening up again. Part of the reality of trust is earned by listening with sensitivity and genuine caring. The quality of listening is a vital component of trust. Taking constant notes of what I am saying has to be done very skilfully if I am to believe that genuine listening and caring is taking place. Sometimes this works but often it does not. Being faced by someone with a blank sheet of paper to fill can leave me feeling unsettled and cautious.

We (patients) do not talk to vicariously write our thoughts and experiences, but because we need help, and want to believe the person we are talking to can actually offer that help. My psychiatrist writes down just about everything I say, and that is OK because I trust him now. But it took a long time to establish this trust, which developed as a result of my experience of his decision-making which I could clearly see the wisdom of, even if just in retrospect.

The other aspect of trust is that the patient has to know that the person they are confiding in and working with is strong enough to deal with the issues without it distressing them. Or at the very least that they have in place somewhere to take issues that may arise that they may find difficult. I have, on more than one occasion been offered help, only to discover that these lines of support were not in place and my artwork in particular caused a lot of distress to the people concerned. For obvious reasons I felt guilty for 'overloading' them, whereas it has been pointed out since that the problem was not mine but belonged to the other person involved. Now if I have any doubts I check this out with the professional before establishing a therapeutic relationship. I am not alone in being worried about this sort of problem. A great number of fellow patients I have met and come to know over the years share this very concern. (It is my belief that the *degree* of depression suffered by many highly sensitive people results from their heightened sensitivity making them more than usually vulnerable to stresses of this kind.)

Being given the real opportunity to express myself

This means someone cares about taking the time to listen and allowing me the time to express myself. This includes allowing me the time and space to talk about my art work and what it is about, or 'just' to talk, or taking the time to read my written work, such as my case word paintings. (A word painting is my expression to describe a painting in language, similar to a poem, of my experience or feelings. Often I start with the raw emotion and through the course of writing the word painting I reach some sort of resolution so that what started as unsafe becomes once more a place of safety for me. There are two examples of word paintings later in this chapter.)

Appropriate, intelligent comment that leads into interactive creativity is most helpful once my contribution has been given the attention and space it warrants as being part of me. So often my artwork is met with blank looks, even when I try and explain it. The *'listener'* isn't really interested or thinks they will never understand because my work is abstract and they describe themselves as 'not at all artistic'. Thus they set themselves up for failure before even beginning to look at my work. Acceptance of what I have to offer and bring to the appointment has to be a primary basis of the listener–patient relationship. (Actually, my artwork is very simple to understand if I am given the opportunity to explain it.)

An example is given below. When I created this particular image (the first in a series), I felt that the poppy represented a facet of myself well: my personal past conflicts and losses (prompted by and reflective of poppy fields/remembrance). The association for me was not with the poppy's natural beauty, but with its association with global conflict.

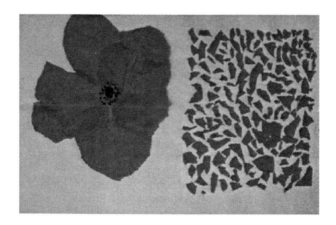

The torn tissue paper 'box' represented my sense of fragmented self that was a consequence of this conflict, and an important source of my ill-health. After a period of reflection, both on my own and with professionals, I was able to clarify in my mind the specific relevance of the poppy image, and the fact that the completed image as a whole was not unattractive. Indeed it could be seen as a positive image, just as the end result of the process of completing these images could be seen as positive.

It may be helpful to clarify the *process* of producing an image that I tend to go through. First, I see in my mind's eye the finished image or part of it. At this stage I have no real conscious insight or understanding of its meaning, just a clear image or part image in my mind. Next, I produce the image using whatever medium seems most appropriate. Whilst working on it the relevance and earliest insights begin to emerge. The final stages are to talk through the image and its meaning to me with a professional, and to leave the image out in my room so that I can live with it and begin to make connections between it, and aspects of my life past and present.

It is thus very important that the time spent with a professional is suitably reflective, questioning, positive and revealing – 'uncovering the layers' within the image and revealing what lies behind it. While I may know in my mind the actual conflict that sparked the image, I have found it helpful to avoid looking for 'a cause' of the conflict itself. Instead, I try to focus on the process of *experiencing and resolving* the conflict. In this image for example, alongside the image of the poppy, the process of using torn tissue paper was very significant for me, as was the idea of containment of the fragments 'in a box' as it were, and the careful tearing and placing of each piece of tissue paper.

In working with this image, the process as a whole allowed me to explore:

1. the (for me) ambiguous beautiful/painful image (poppy) and its resonance with my view of myself
2. a process of fragmentation of my 'self' as a consequence of my experiences
3. a process of recovery whereby I am able to marshal these fragments into a sense of order and containment

Being given the space to talk about the here and now

This is different from the above in that the above is usually structured, prepared time given by appointment and planned for in advance (by me, if not the professional involved). Of course any well trained and experienced professional will keep themselves in a state of readiness to cope with whatever comes their way during working hours. It is hoped that a few seconds/minutes will be taken before the appointment to 'put away' the last task and focus on the next. One of the most helpful times for me was the occasion when I kept my appointment out of politeness, only to say that I was feeling suicidal and didn't think I could cope with talking about something as challenging as abstract art, however relevant it may be (this being our shared brief). The response I got surprised me. It was: 'OK then, come through and talk about suicide.' (I had expected to be let off the hook and be sent back to the ward!)

Talking about suicide that day was really helpful. It didn't stop me feeling suicidal but it made me think more carefully about the contents of my suicide notes and their inadequacy. I went back to the ward intent upon re-thinking the ones I had written and re-writing them so the recipients would find them more supportive. This required real concentration and eventually I fell asleep to awake in a more positive frame of mind with the intention of trying to hang on an hour at a time throughout the day if I possibly could.

Any patient would tell you that whereas the planned appointment is helpful there are always some times when focussing on what is happening in the immediacy of the moment is what is needed. My experience has been that while some professionals recognise this there are all too many who want to know **why** I feel like this (**past**) and how to move on (**future**) without ever looking at or accepting the fact that this is where I am *NOW.*

Interactive creativity

The emphasis being here is on both interactive *and* creativity. I often use metaphor in my description of how things are and I find it really helpful if the 'listener' can paraphrase my statements in an equally creative manner. For example I may say: "it feels as if I am being sucked down a drain". A helpful response for me at such a point would incorporate one or more of the following constituent parts: the fact I am going down, that this is not in my control, and that it is a decidedly unpleasant experience. Maybe a bit like falling from a great height and one is totally at the mercy of gravity, or other analogies showing understanding. Such responses would give me the opportunity of agreeing or disagreeing and possibly a mutual exploration of possible images until we find one that more exactly describes how I am feeling. This empowers me because by being able to identify my emotions very exactly puts me back in ownership and closer to control.

Words are very approximate for the best of us and it is only by 'feeling around' for the right image or set of ideas that we may be more precise about our feelings. Just stop for a minute and identify the feelings you have had this morning – I bet you found either a lot of imagery or a very limited vocabulary. Looking behind that vocabulary, taking it apart and rebuilding it with a wider panorama is *really* helpful. The act of listening and acknowledging the aptness of the description is very important. So, too, is the development of ideas through interactive creative thinking, for then the patient knows they are part of a process that demands the attention of both participants. As a shared commitment to the recovery process, creative thinking is, in my experience *always* helpful if done with another person, but may not be accessible to a person on their own if they are feeling particularly low or slowed down by drugs.

Positive, active silence

Silence can convey so much when two people are together, preferably interacting. It can, for instance convey criticism, judgement, empathy, creativity, or even simple acceptance, or non-acceptance.

Active, shared silence is negotiated between two people and conveyed by facial expression, attention, and body language. Vulnerable people are extremely sensitive to such signals, and will, if possible, interpret them negatively. Therefore there should be little ambiguity. Acceptance and a shared experience of each silence and its purpose is possible and can be powerfully helpful. When to use such silences has to be instinctive and open, but need not be approached verbally. It needs to be a relevant part of the process. It allows space for thought, and reflection of what has gone before and maybe what is to follow. Sharing real, vital issues is a draining and exhausting process for both parties, but particularly for the patient who may be sharing what to them, is a real horror story, even if 'just' talking about the events of the last hour or two.

Consistency and co-operation

When I am being supported in the community, I am very lucky to work within a team of committed, creative workers who work together with me to ensure the service I receive is consistent and meets my needs. This is not only done very effectively through the CPA process but through internal communication within the team so everyone knows where I am at and can fulfil their particular role within my circle of complex needs. I am, and always feel, an integral part of the team. We work together – that means I work at least as hard as they do at moving on and/or consolidation as required at any given moment. Roles are clearly agreed and we all stick within our own boundaries.

Unfortunately the same cannot yet be said of all my experiences within a hospital setting. This is partly my own fault because if one nurse suggests something that I find unhelpful, rather than going back and challenging the nurse with an update, it is so much easier to talk to another nurse. This avoids hurting the feelings of the first nurse and allows for the creativity of the subsequent nurses I may speak to. This is very unfair to the nurses and assumes they don't talk to each other about problems individual patients may be experiencing on their shift. This is clearly nonsense and naïve, but nevertheless many patients behave this way. Feeling vulnerable (which one does in hospital) is daunting, if not frightening, and to go back to a nurse, or other professional (who are perceived as being very powerful people) and challenge them, however gently, on the advice they have given is testing. The following extract from something I wrote when I was last discharged sums up my experience in this sense:

> "One hell of a place – all bustling and chatter and power games.
> Do this – go there
> remember to remind us to give you your medication.
> Go to bed,
> try to sleep,
> have a pill and try again.
> Stay in your room,
> get out of your room,
> mix with others,
> take time out,
> keep busy,
> have a rest,
> go for a walk,

try hugging a tree.
Listen to this relaxation tape,
come to this stress management class.
Hospital – so much for asylum.
No connection in my mind.
But then what is my mind?
A jumble of mixed up,
confused thoughts.
Can't think why!"

Safety

The concept of safety is of paramount importance. For me this means staying in control of my emotions even as I express them. One particularly helpful technique has been to give me a very limited time (in a recent situation, I was 'given' 30 seconds!) to express feelings or even facts, knowing that it will be contained in that time and the boundaries are very clear. It also means safety in that I know that the person I am sharing my thoughts and feelings can cope with them and not get distressed by them. Their strength is vital to me. My word paintings when shared have, on occasion in the past, caused real distress to the professional I was sharing them with. This in turn made it unsafe for me to continue.

It is not that I am unwilling to talk, or to be guided in sharing what I am ready and able to share. This comes down both to trust and personal responsibility. I am responsible for what I say, but often a conversation can trigger a particularly difficult set of thoughts some time later, leaving me feeling as described in the word painting above.

The following word painting was written nine years ago, and is a poignant reminder of the importance of safety in any therapeutic work.

You find one,
You test it out.
It stands the test,
so you test it a little harder.
So slowly you learn to trust,
to feel safe there,
safe places are like people.
Then suddenly,
even there,
you are invaded in the depths

Of your most private being,
and stripped of all structure,
and you have to start
All over again.
Trusting is so hard.
It makes no difference
how carefully you build
the barriers,
how slyly you work out
where people will look,
where they are least likely to pry
or to peep.
How carefully
you prepare the ground,
you can never outwit
The bully with brains.
And so you are left
trembling with terror,
full of fury,
and hurting with such deep,
deep, pain, that when they are gone –
even then,
all you are left with
is the pain of the knowing
how stupid you were
to try and trust,
or to hide,
to find a safe place
through the sorrow filled
corridors of silent sadness,
trying to trust,
trying anything,
anything at all that might
help with the horror.
And hoping,
hoping so hard
for an end to it all.

(14.1.94)

Conclusion

Strength, gentleness and genuine caring are the three essentials that I look for in the professionals with whom I work. I am privileged to work with a team of just such people. My understanding of the Consultant Nurse function is that these qualities are valid interpretations of the Department of Health's wishes of the role, as seen in the '4 key functions' of the Consultant Nurse (DoH, 1999). Strength is about providing safety, both at an individual and organisational level – modelling sound practice and exerting influence in healthcare circles to improve the capacity of the system to be safe and *feel* safe to vulnerable people. Gentleness refers to the hope that these most senior nurses will recall the origins, the nurturing, compassion and caring arts upon which nursing is based – and resist the temptation to become remote or distant from the patient because of 'expertness'. Finally, genuine caring is a quality that no one can feign. The patient will always be able to discriminate between the truly caring Consultant Nurse and those who pretend.

Index